Palliative Care for People with AIDS

SECOND EDITION

Ruth Sims RGN, DNCert, Dip NAMH
Chief Executive
Mildmay Mission Hospital
London

Veronica A Moss MB BS, DTM&H,
DCH, DObst RCOG
Medical Director
Mildmay Mission Hospital
London

Edward Arnold
A member of the Hodder Headline Group
LONDON   SYDNEY   AUCKLAND

First published in Great Britain 1991 as *Terminal Care for People with AIDS*
Second edition published 1995 by
Edward Arnold, a division of Hodder Headline PLC,
338 Euston Road, London NW1 3BH

British Library Cataloguing in Publication Data
A catalogue record for this book is available from the British Library

ISBN 0 340 61371 8

5 4 3 2 1   99 98 97 96 95

Typeset in 9.5/11 Palatino by
York House Typographic Ltd, London
Printed and bound in Great Britain by
J W Arrowsmith Ltd, Bristol

To all those people with AIDS whom
we have come to know and love,
and especially to those who have
lived with us at Mildmay.

Contents

Foreword to the second edition

The global pandemic of AIDS and HIV infection continues to escalate in all countries in which this disease has been reported. The WHO estimate (in 1993) that by the year 2000, up to 13 million people will have AIDS, and up to 40 million people will have been infected with HIV. In the United Kingdom, 9,436 AIDS diagnoses had been reported by the end of June 1994 and 22,101 had been confirmed HIV-1 positive.

AIDS is today the greatest threat to the public health in our life-time and has presented us with unique challenges. For the caring professions, these challenges have most frequently focused on the need to offer competent, confident and compassionate care for those thousands of often frightened individuals requiring medical and nursing support. To do this effectively, health care professionals need an opportunity to extend their skills and knowledge, and space to explore their own attitudes to the highly charged issues which AIDS demands we confront. One of the most difficult issues requiring exploration is our response to death and dying.

Death is part of life and dying is simply 'living the end of life'. My own experience in caring for people with AIDS has reminded me of the common wish we all have to 'live the end of our life' well. To support patients with AIDS 'living the end of their life' well requires skill and an awareness of the unique needs of individuals nearing that end. These include the needs to be safe and not to be hurt, to be given refuge or sanctuary, to be comforted and accepted, to belong, and to give and receive love.

This important book is about meeting those needs. It is not about death but about 'living the end of our life' well. It describes a unique model of care which has been created by Ruth Sims, Veronica Moss and their colleagues at a rather special hospital in the East End of London. The on-going dynamic experiences of the Mildmay Mission Hospital are charting a path through our fears and confusion in relation to offering quality care to individuals seeking support for an appropriate end to their life.

It describes a sensitive and comprehensive approach to the practical issues involved in meeting the terminal care needs of individuals with AIDS. Like its authors, this book reflects love and hope and provides for the first time the expert guidance needed to be with our patients in a meaningful way as they confront the final stage of their lives.

We are all going to have the experience, many times over before this epidemic has run its course, of knowing and loving individuals 'living the end of their life' with AIDS. This book shows us how to do it and I commend it to all health care professionals.

Robert J. Pratt RN, BA, MSc, RGN, RNT, DipN(Lond).
Vice Principal/Head of Faculty
Faculty of Continuing Education
Riverside College of Nursing, London
1994

Acknowledgements

Many people have helped and encouraged us in the writing of this book and we would like them to know how much their encouragement has been appreciated.

In particular Robert Pratt, Vice Principal, The Riverside College of Nursing of London, without whose encouragement and advice this book would probably never have been written, and Mrs Taylor-Thompson, the Chairman of the Mildmay Board of Directors, who, from the very beginning, has been entirely enthusiastic and supportive in our venture.

A number of colleagues and friends who should have special mention have encouraged us and given advice related to their particular speciality: Shirley Lunn, Head of Counselling and Welfare, Rev. Peter Clarke, Director of Chaplaincy Services, both at Mildmay since the beginning of the AIDS work; John Atkinson in Glasgow; Dr Ray Brettle and Dr Jacqueline Mok in Edinburgh; Professor A. Pinching and Dr Jane Anderson at St Bartholomew's Hospital, London; Dr Di Gibb and Candy Duggan at the Hospital for Sick Children, Great Ormond Street, London; Richard Wells, former Head of Rehabilitation, Royal Marsden Hospital, and former AIDS Adviser to the World Health Organisation; our many friends who have AIDS, in particular Peter Tillson and Kevin Rimington from whom we have learnt so much. We also want to thank the Terence Higgins Trust, ACET, Positively Women, Grandma's and Christopher Spence of the London Lighthouse.

We are grateful to the many people who have given us invaluable advice and information relating to developing countries and areas where resources for care are more limited than in Britain. Special mention must be made of the following people with whom we have met or worked: Mrs Esther Gatua, Director of HIV/AIDS Projects, Christian Health Association of Kenya; Mrs Ndorito, Chief Nurse, Kenya Catholic Secretariat; Mrs Kimeni, Kenya's Adviser to the WHO; Mrs Gitei, Kenya AIDS Control Programme; Mrs Oduri, Chief Nurse of Kenya; Dr Miriam Duggan, Nsambya Hospital, Uganda; Sister Agatha Sembuye,

Namirembe Diocesan Counsellor and AIDS project planner, Church of Uganda; Sr Ursula, Kitovu Hospital, Uganda; Dr James Makumbi the Minister of Health for Uganda; Hon. Manuel Pinto, Director of Uganda AIDS Commission; the Minister of Health for Zimbabwe, Dr T. Stamp; Professor Latif, Parirenyatua Hospital, Harare, and Dr Geoff Forster, Paediatrician, Mutare Provincial Hospital, Zimbabwe.

Many others from other areas of the world have contributed to our understanding, including Captain Ian Campbell, Medical Adviser to the Salvation Army, the doctor responsible for implementing an integrated AIDS Care and Counselling Home Care programme from Chikankata Hospital, Zambia, and Professor A. Bailey, Zambia. Discussion with our numerous visitors from many parts of the world, including Eastern Bloc countries, Asia and North and South America, have widened our horizons and sharpened our appreciation of the many challenges facing the world regarding the issues around HIV/AIDS. Last but not least, we have learnt from our many patients from all parts of the world.

Finally, we would like to thank all staff at Mildmay for their support. We are grateful especially to the non-executive and executive directors; and to our secretaries for their very practical support and hard work in preparing the original manuscripts and now again with the new edition. We are grateful to them for their patience in dealing with corrections and alterations while continuing to perform their other duties with their usual efficiency.

Notes to readers

Gender The person with AIDS may be a man, woman or child, but for ease of reference the words he or him rather than the more cumbersome he/she or him/her have been used throughout this book.

Family Included in the term 'family' is anyone who is important to the patient – a partner, anyone related by blood or marriage, or a close friend. By partner we mean the person to whom the patient has the deepest commitment: the one who is acknowledged as the present partner is the one nominated by the patient as such. It may therefore refer to a husband, a wife, a common law husband or wife, or a lover.

Counsellor This word is used to refer to anyone who has a training in counselling and who has formal commitments to the work of counselling. This may refer to a social worker with counselling remit, or a psychologist as well as to the person who has a recognised training in counselling.

This book is *not*
- a text book on AIDS
- a text book on how to be a counsellor, how to nurse etc.
- a book about education or prevention of AIDS

This book does not pretend to have all the answers. It does not try to deal with any subjects that are outside our experience. It is a book which simply seeks to share the experience and understanding gained during the past seven years from talking with, working with, and living with people with AIDS. Much time has also been spent talking with and learning from other health care professionals involved in the care of people with AIDS in Britain and abroad. Most of what we write is of our own personal experience; but none of it has been in isolation from the rest of the team. For all in the multiprofessional team at Mildmay it has been a time of learning together. Of course there is still much to be learnt.

This book does not enter into issues related to politics or debates about lifestyles We do not believe that the terminal care arena is appropriate for such debate. Suffice it to say that we believe that no person should be discriminated against in any way; all are deserving of the highest standards of care, given with genuine love and acceptance, and backed by sufficient funding and manpower to enable each person living with AIDS to do so with dignity and in the place of his choice.

'Patients' Our consumer research indicated that people with AIDS in our care setting were comfortable with the term 'patient'. They were familiar with it as recipients of care in hospitals or the community and saw no reason to be called anything else.

Abbreviations

Abbreviations used in this book (see in particular Chapter 6)

Dosages and administration of drugs

bd	twice daily; alternatively bid
BM	bowel movement
4 hourly	to be taken every 4 hours; alt. q4h
h	hour(s)
IM	intramuscular
IV	intravenous
kg	kilogram
l	litre
lb	pound
mg	milligram(s)
ml	millilitre(s)
mm	millimetre(s)
mmol	millimole(s)
min	minute(s)
μg	microgram(s)
NSAID	non-steroidal anti-inflammatory drug(s)
nocte	at night
od	once daily
po	per os; by mouth
pr	per rectum
prn	pro re nata, 'as required'
qds	four times in 24 hours; alt. qid
s-c	sub cutaneous
sl	sub lingual
stat	at once
tds	three times in 24 hours; alt. tid

Introduction

Why a book on terminal care for people with AIDS?

Much has been written in recent years both on terminal care in general and on AIDS in particular. The general principles of terminal care, as practised in traditional hospices and through such home support services as those provided by Macmillan nurses, are well established. Knowledge about AIDS and of how it takes its inexorable toll on human lives, is growing day by day. So is there a need for a book which deals with terminal care and AIDS?

We believe that there is such a need. The advent of AIDS has challenged science to find answers very quickly. In the major cities of Great Britain, most general practitioners now have at least one or two persons with HIV or AIDS on their books, most district nurses have had some experience of nursing someone with AIDS at home, many midwives and health visitors are becoming familiar with issues around HIV/AIDS in pregnancy and childhood. It is still true that many community carers in other parts of Britain have not yet faced that challenge, but they will have to do so, sooner or later. Many people already know someone whose life has been touched by bereavement through AIDS. In America and in many developing countries as well as in Britain, increasing numbers of women and children, whole families and communities are being affected.

When compared with deaths caused by other modern 'epidemics', such as road traffic accidents, heart disease and cervical cancer, the number of deaths resulting from AIDS is still relatively small. However, when the rapid spread to date and the frightening prevalence rates that are now being reported in the USA and in many parts of the Third World are considered it is clear that there is no room for complacency.

This is particularly true when considering young heterosexual people who have, in the main, not accepted the need for changes in the attitudes to casual sex that have been part of Western culture since the 1960s. It is even more true when thinking about those who are addicted

Table i. Common features of AIDS which are likely to differ from those of the terminally ill patient with cancer

---

1. Predominantly younger age group (0–5 years; 16–49 years).
2. Multisystems disease with multiple problems:
   - blindness
   - paralysis
   - neuropathy
   - dementia
   - myopathy
   - skin disorders
   - severe diarrhoea
   - chest infections.
3. Misery of many co-existing diagnoses.
4. Polypharmacy.
5. Sudden, dramatic changes in condition – difficulty in identification of terminal phase.
6. Need for very active palliation or maintenance, e.g. with IV infusions and treatment of opportunistic infections.
7. Lengthy dying process – at times patients may be unconscious for a week or more.
8. Changing pattern of disease and treatment.
9. Patient awareness relating to the disease and its treatment.
10. Isolation, stigma and lack of compassion for patient and family.
11. Lack of family and support structures.
12. Housing problems including homelessness, inappropriate accommodation and need for supervision.

---

to drugs who often take double risks – sexually and through the sharing of needles.

There is also a need to dispel some of the fears and prejudices that are still so evident among some health care professionals. Many others are prepared and willing to get involved, but are apprehensive of the unknown. There are many similarities in the terminal care required for people with cancer and that required for those with AIDS. However there are also major differences (see Table i) which we hope to clarify.

Our aims

In writing this book we aim to increase the awareness of health care professionals to the issues surrounding terminal care for people with AIDS. We hope this will enable them to make more appropriate responses to the needs of those who come to them for help. We hope, too, that the practical guidelines given will enable them to make those responses with confidence. The practical guidelines and general principles are based on the experience we have gained during the past seven years. Since January 1987 we have been responsible for researching, planning, and establishing Europe's first AIDS hospice and continuing care unit at Mildmay in the East End of London. This includes day and home care provided by a multiprofessional team. We have learnt most from those who are living with AIDS – many of whom have been our patients. We have also learnt much from their families, friends and partners. We have witnessed tremendous courage and devotion, and have felt the challenge to re-examine our practice and attitudes in relation to all client groups. We pass this challenge on to you.

1

Where to care

In the United Kingdom the options available for the terminal care of people with AIDS fall into two main categories:

- *hospital care*
- *community care,* i.e.
    home care
    sheltered accommodation
    hospice care
    day care.

Care in the hospital

At the present time the majority of people with AIDS who need care choose to be cared for by staff at designated AIDS centres in major cities. The reasons for this are many but include:

- the belief that the very best in care is provided only at these centres
- there they will be accepted and need not fear the rejection and prejudice associated with their diagnosis
- they can preserve their anonymity in a way which they could not do if using local services.

Despite the increase in numbers of people with AIDS this is still the case, especially in London. Beds in designated AIDS wards are full, and often as many patients as are in the ward are disseminated throughout the same hospital into general wards, under the care of the consultant in HIV disease. This would account for the fact that many health care professionals working outside of major cities may never have met or cared for a person with AIDS, indeed they will have seen nothing of the reality of the growing demand for services.

A recent survey has shown that the majority of people with AIDS still die in hospital (Kennedy, 1990). For many patients, especially those

who have had repeated hospital admissions, this is entirely appropriate. The security of being cared for in familiar surroundings by people
who may have known the patient since he was first diagnosed, and who
clearly care for and about the patient, cannot be underestimated. For
some people the maintenance of hope that comes of being in an acute
care setting is essential if living, for them, is to have quality. For others
the availability of emergency treatment, if needed, helps to allay fears.

What is community care?

Is it being at home with family who care about you and are prepared to
give that caring practical expression, asking for very little outside help?

Is it home care given mainly by professionals and volunteers with
input from friends and family?

Or is it similar to the following experience.

A young man lives alone in his London flat refusing all care
save the help of his buddy. AIDS has been scored in the wood
of his front door – it is sad to see the desperate, unsuccessful
attempts he has made to obliterate it. He refuses to go out for
fear he will be attacked. He is not receiving care from statutory
services; he is afraid of who might be sent to care for him.

He has experienced so much rejection and persecution that
he just cannot risk it again.

Sadly, there are people, including health care professionals, who would
justify these very fears.

In providing appropriate terminal care it is essential to identify needs:
needs as perceived by the patient and those important to him. Provision
and choice of care should therefore be in response to those needs. In
order to identify needs it is essential to involve patients, giving them
relevant information and choices. It should be remembered that many
people in the terminal stages of the disease will be suffering from
dementia; whenever possible in the planning of care, options should be
presented to the patient and those important to him, and liaisons
established as early as possible.

The Government White Paper 'Caring for people' describes community care in the following way:

Community care means providing the right level of intervention and
support to enable people to achieve maximum independence and
control over their own lives. For this aim to become a reality, the
development of a wide range of services provided in a variety of
settings is essential.

Care in the community

Bill was 32 years of age. He was a person with AIDS living in San Francisco – and he was dying. At over six feet tall he was painfully thin, weighing only a few stones. He looked like an old man, emaciated and balding.

I first met Bill in a small dark room in what I can only describe as a broken down hotel. The curtains were pinned together at the window and Bill was wearing dark glasses. Everything was dark and dismal. A kitten was jumping around the room, as were fleas, and there were cockroaches on the table and in cupboards. Bill was huddled in his bed looking wretched.

I saw many patients in similar surroundings in San Francisco. Would they not have been much happier in the airy light and comfortable surroundings of the Coming Home residential hospice?

For them, I was told, it would not have been better. The thing Bill valued most was his independence, the ability to control his own life and surroundings, to make decisions and to retain his dignity. His experience was that this was in no way possible to any similar extent in any care-providing institution.

In spite of living in squalor, community care was right for Bill.

Martin was 24 years of age. He was a person with AIDS – he was dying.

He had occupied an acute bed in a London hospital for several weeks and the decision was made that he should be discharged to his parents' home where they would care for him. Martin had not lived with them for seven years. They could not handle the fact that he was gay, especially as they did not want him, as they put it, influencing his two younger brothers and turning them 'that way'. He had lived for the past four years with his partner John, who had cared for him in the flat they shared prior to Martin's admission to hospital. John had not been allowed any input into the decision made regarding Martin's discharge and Martin was too weak to fight his parents.

When Martin went to the family home he was emaciated, incontinent of urine and faeces, had oral and oesophageal candida and was thoroughly wretched and depressed. He was very withdrawn and spoke very little.

The statutory and voluntary services were called in with input from the general practitioner, District Nursing Services, Social Services (home help) and Crossroads Care Attendant Scheme. His nursing care was excellent, his symptom control good and voluntary help enabled his parents to cope. His parents, however, were concerned that his two younger brothers be protected both from Martin and his lifestyle. John was never allowed to visit their home.

Martin died after ten days, without the love and support of the person who mattered most in the world to him.

For Martin, although input from statutory and voluntary services was good, some of his most fundamental needs were not met and community care was not best for him.

Care at home

Care at home involves caring for the patient and those important to him as a unit. When it is successful, care provided in the familiar surroundings of the home, with multiprofessional input from the statutory and voluntary services, can produce the very best of terminal care. In the freedom of their own homes independence is often more easily maintained and people can behave as they wish. When home care is the appropriate option it should be available and accessible to everyone who needs it.

Care in sheltered accommodation

For people who are increasingly facing homelessness and are chronically ill but still self caring and not requiring nursing care, there is a great need for sheltered accommodation. At the present time this need remains unfulfilled in England except for a very few initiatives. Provision is being planned in some areas by voluntary organisations, private individuals and by housing associations. A number of these are also seeking to provide homes for people in the form of flats or rooms within houses.

In this situation supervision is often necessary, with a 'warden' or person on call, as is the provision of one hot meal per day. Special accommodation may not be required. The clients have similar needs to any chronically sick person, but the diagnosis of AIDS may result in rejection from general provision.

The provision of sheltered accommodation for people with AIDS is an identified gap in service provision, especially in areas such as London where there are large numbers of people with AIDS who require care.

Care in a hospice

For some patients, hospice care will be the most appropriate, whether it be in a traditional hospice or a designated unit such as the Mildmay or London Lighthouse. The circumstances include when:

- the patient is living alone
- there is poor symptom control
- there are frightening symptoms.

Hospices will need to be able to offer 24 hour multiprofessional care. *Time* for patients, time to care, time to listen or just time to 'be there'; this can only be achieved with high staffing ratios.

The advantages of hospice care include:

- living in a homely setting
- the privacy of a private room but the opportunity to share communal facilities
- continuing care including respite, rehabiliative and convalescent care, referral back to acute centres and support and counselling for partners and families
- bereavement support and follow up.

Day care facilities

The aims of providing a non acute day care facility as part of the continuum of care are:

- to enable people to remain at home for as long as possible
- to enhance the quality of life of patients and their carers.

To achieve this the care on offer should include:

- treatment facilities
  palliative and maintenance only
  assistance with bathing and personal care
  emotional support and counselling
  dental treatment
  chiropody
  rehabilitation including physiotherapy, occupational and art therapies, massage, etc.
- provision of hot meals
- welfare advice and help

- respite for patient and/or carer
- recreational facilities
  films, concerts, visiting artistes
  crafts
  hairdressing.

'Traditional' hospices offering day care may make their facilities available to people with AIDS.

Having looked at the options for care and what they offer, what are the possible problems relating to these options?

Problems with hospital care

Understaffing and the high dependency of patients in the acute hospital may make it difficult for carers to have time to look after people in the way that they would like. Input to the families, partners and friends of the patient in terms of support, help and counselling is usually limited. Bereavement support and counselling is often non-existent. Many patients with AIDS are in need of terminal care for weeks or even months with resultant pressures on staff and on the demand for beds.

Problems with community care

Problems with home care

Can 24 hour care be provided when it is needed? In the United Kingdom it has seldom been possible to provide 24 hour care for patients other than for those suffering from advanced malignant disease, and then demand for services has far exceeded supply. Can spans of care for 4–8 hours be provided to enable the primary carer to go out to work? Are district nurses trained and ready to give the intravenous (IV) drugs and total parenteral nutrition becoming more and more necessary in palliative care for people with AIDS? Who will give the tremendous input of skilled counselling needed by these patients and those they love? Can bereavement support and follow up be provided to families at home?

Problems with care in sheltered accommodation

At present people living in sheltered accommodation are not always linked with local statutory and voluntary services, resulting in problems when residents become acutely ill or when those with chronic illness need skilled nursing rather than supervisory care. Planners of care need to ensure that, at the very least, there is an informed and sympathetic general practitioner who is willing to take the residents on to his or her list. It is encouraging that in some areas of London planners of hostels and halfway houses are involved in joint planning committees, liaising with and developing local services.

Problems with hospice care

For some patients hospice care may be unacceptable. For some it signifies the end of the line: 'No more can be done, everyone has given up on me'. This option must be presented with considerable sensitivity. Hospices offering respite and convalescent care help to allay fears that people admitted to a hospice are there only to die.

Many traditional hospices, that is those caring mainly for patients with cancer, are either unable or unwilling to admit people with AIDS. The reasons for non-acceptance include:

- funding is/has been given only for patients with cancer
- inadequate facilities; unable to cope with demand for beds from people with cancer
- insufficient medical cover
- management level decision
- hospice staff unwilling or feel unqualified to care for people with AIDS.

Whatever the reason given, the outcome is that there are patients travelling miles from home to receive care that could much more appropriately be given nearer their home.

Wherever the care is offered the *aim* should be the same – *to give care that is responsive to the total needs of the patient and his family, i.e. physical, emotional, spiritual and social needs*. All carers share the same concerns. With hospitals and hospital wards closing in the UK the pressure on acute beds is increasing. This results in earlier discharge of patients into the community without proportionate transfer of funding and resources. This, together with the earlier discharge of post-operative patients, patients from acute elderly rehabilitation wards, and the emphasis on community care for the disabled, is causing overstretching and under-funding of community services, with inevitable low morale and understaffing. This could result in diluted services and have a devastating effect on the quality and range of community care.

Many areas are tackling the problem, setting up educational programmes and support for staff, liaising, appointing advisors and/or specialist teams, researching need and investigating new initiatives. There remains, however, much to be done if we are to be able to offer options, real choices, for care to the projected numbers of people with AIDS who will die in this country this century.

Mark's story

Mark was in his early twenties. He came with his mother to 'have a look round' before deciding whether he wanted to be admitted to Mildmay. He was referred for 'terminal care'. Mark had ideally wanted to stay at home but that was not possible as his mother and father worked and he was too frightened to spend long periods of time alone. He decided he would come to Mildmay and was admitted the next day. He was suffering from peripheral neuropathy and atypical mycobacterial disease.

Within 24 hours of admission Mark developed a severe abdominal pain and the team felt that he should be offered the opportunity of returning to his acute centre for investigations and possible surgery. Having been made comfortable, Mark was seen by the doctor and his primary nurse who discussed with him the options and likely outcomes. He asked if he could have two hours to decide and requested that the local Roman Catholic parish priest (a man not known to him) visit him. He talked with the priest and was given the last rites. At 4 pm Mark told the team that he had decided that he wished to have no further acute interventions. He knew that he may die quite soon but that was his choice and he told his parents of his decision. Over a period of 24 hours it seemed that this young boy had become a man.

Mark did not die; in fact, he lived for a year – his condition stabilised and, for a time, he improved a great deal. This time was very important to him and his parents, a time during which they, with the help of the counsellor and the whole multiprofessional team, worked through painful issues and emerged with an openness and honesty that they as a family had never known before.

Mark never lost sight of his wish to die at home. His mother felt guilty that she was out at work and felt unable to care for him at home. However, Mark decided he would like to be at home during weekends. This was arranged with attention to detail so that the whole family felt supported and had adequate back-up. Then Mark developed cytomegalovirus (CMV) retinitis – he had dreaded this possibility because, apart from the deteriorating vision, he was needle phobic.

Mark again looked at his options and decided he could not risk going blind, and would therefore opt for having intravenous ganciclovir infusions. He returned to his acute centre to have the Hickman line sited. By now his mother was more confident about his visits home, his relationship with his father was much better and Mark really wanted to spend longer at home. But the infusion . . . his parents felt quite unable to take it on, he would have to go home just for odd days. Community care of his intravenous infusion was not available. Mark took control of the situation – he still wanted to die at home but his condition was deteriorating and he knew this. Needle phobic or not. Mark decided that he would learn to administer his ganciclovir and flush his line. He felt that he needed the freedom to control his environment rather than, as he saw it, having the environment control him. His mother was also taught to give the infusion and gradually they both became more confident. She had decided by now to give up her job so that she could care for Mark at home. The home care nurses visited Mark and his family on the unit and he was glad to establish relationships. His discharge was carefully planned so that he had several trial weekends before finally going home. He regularly contacted the unit to let the team know how he was. His mother cared for him with only the minimum of input from community services. This was as Mark wanted it. After 12 weeks at home Mark died peacefully. His parents were well supported by the home care team and the priest who was now their friend.

Mark did take control of his life. He made choices with outcomes that his family and the staff found difficult and challenging, and overcame tremendous personal fears and obstacles to make his wish to die at home become a reality.

References

Government White Paper (1989), *Caring for People – Community care in the next decade and beyond*. CM 849. HMSO, London.

Kennedy, A. (1990). Communicable Disease Surveillance Centre, Public Health Laboratories. (Unpublished).

2

Responding to the terminal care needs of people with AIDS

People with AIDS have a need to *live* with AIDS, and not just to sit, or lie, around waiting to die. The Oxford English Dictionary describes 'to live' as meaning 'to be alive'. This living can embrace a broad spectrum from, at the one end, a meaningless miserable existence to, at the other end, living with quality.

The Wilkes (1980) report states:

> The main aims of those providing terminal care should be to improve the quality of daily life by removing or alleviating unpleasant symptoms and helping to prevent the patient from suffering fear or loneliness.

'Quality' means different things to different people. Some people enjoy eating whole foods, others enjoy pie and chips. Some people find talking helpful, others find it difficult. People are individuals, all with differing needs; the response to those needs must therefore always be individually tailored.

Who is this person with AIDS whose needs the carer is attempting to address? It is the man, woman, teenager, child or baby who has been referred to the hospital, hospice and/or community services and needs care. The person with AIDS is someone with a multi-systems disease who, in common with all individuals, has needs which must be met if health is to be maintained, needs that must be responded to with quality.

Quality of life can only be maintained and improved if distressing symptoms can be relieved and, recognising the potential that each individual has, working with or for them to maximise this potential. Assumptions about what constitutes quality for individuals should not be made – for some people at certain times quality will mean being allowed to choose to opt out.

Physical needs

As AIDS is a multi-systems disease, its presentation in terminal care is varied and often complex. The patient in the advanced stages of the disease may be ulcerated from mouth to anus with difficulty in eating and swallowing. He may be emaciated, having torrential diarrhoea of several litres a day. He will be weak and tired and may look prematurely old, displaying purple skin lesions over many parts of his body.

The physical care of these patients presents great challenges to carers, not least the need for good clinical management. The problems commonly encountered are:

- total body pain
- neuropathy
- myopathy
- weight loss, often as much as one-third of body weight
- dyspnoea
- nausea and/or vomiting
- diarrhoea
- skin lesions
- severe debility and decreased mobility
- intermittent confusion and inability to maintain personal safety.

Responding to physical needs

AIDS commonly affects people at a time in their life when they would have been at their most creative and productive.

It is essential to work *with* the patient and important that, whenever possible, control is where it belongs – with the patient. Prior to admission many patients will have been cared for by their partner or a family member. It is essential that the partner and/or family member is encouraged to continue to be a key member of the caring team if they and the patient wish it, and provided they are not needing respite themselves.

In order to give control to the patient it is necessary to give information relating to options available. This places considerable responsibility on carers in an area of care which is constantly changing and developing. Having encouraged the patient to make choices it is essential that his wishes are respected. This can be difficult for some carers who may usually be directive in their approach.

It could be argued that for too long care professionals have not listened to their patients; care professionals *alone* have been the assessors, and the care given based on their assessment.

A friend of mine, who is a doctor, was admitted to hospital for major surgery. Less than 24 hours post operatively he asked for an injection as he had severe pain. He was told, 'It can't be that bad yet, you only had an injection 2 hours ago.'

Pain, nausea and discomfort should be as the patient feels it, not as the doctor or nurse thinks it is or should be.

Patients need comfort, that is the physical freedom from discomfort. The response of a multiprofessional team of carers is the best way to achieve this.

Highly skilled medical care must be provided, with input from the doctor as necessary, often on a daily basis. To maintain symptom control (see Chapter 6) it may be necessary to resort to polypharmacy in order to control the many distressing symptoms the patient may have. It may be difficult for doctors in general practice to keep up this level of care for more than one or two terminally ill people at a time, especially over long periods of time. Good symptom control is dependent on effective communication between doctors and nurses (see also Chapter 3).

Highly skilled nursing care with attention to detail is essential. Sometimes the nurse's role is to encourage, sometimes to 'push' a little, but always to be there when needed. Patients need to maintain their independence and skill is required to offer help without pressurising and to give choices, space and time to the patient. Some patients may refuse care and in these cases their wishes must be respected; this may be difficult for the nurse to accept and will often have implications for carers, partners, family and friends. Nurses must know about the disease, its treatment and issues relating to research. Many of the patients will know more about the disease than those caring for them and they will need to discuss issues with their carers. The nurses' skill, knowledge, attitudes and standards of care must give them credibility with their patients (see also Chapter 4).

Input from *rehabilitative therapies* is likely to be invaluable in terms of restoring and maintaining physical function.

At times it may be necessary to give treatments not normally given in a terminal care setting, for example the use of

- intravenous ganciclovir (daily or 3–5 days per week is the usual regime) to prevent progression to blindness in patients with cytomegalovirus (CMV) retinitis
- total parenteral nutrition (TPN) to patients with chronic diarrhoea, severe weight loss or swallowing difficulties

● nebulised pentamidine as a prophylaxis against *Pneumocystis carinii* pneumonia fortnightly or monthly.

The above are maintenance therapies initiated in acute centres and, in some areas, the treatments are maintained in the community. When the human immunodeficiency virus affects the brain, the resultant dementia will render increasing numbers of people unable to maintain their own safety and independence. Even in the ideal situation it is impossible to provide literal 24 hour care – the minute you turn your back the patient will fall! There will always be an element of risk which has to be accepted, as the cost to the patient of total safety would surely be unacceptable.

Emotional needs

The emotional environment is created by people interacting with the patient, people demonstrating that they care and showing unconditional love and acceptance (see also Chapter 7). The needs for love, acceptance and security are particularly important in this care setting as many people with AIDS will have experienced rejection for much of their lives. This rejection may have caused them to leave the family home, physically separating themselves from all people, family and 'friends', familiar to them. Loneliness and isolation can be difficult and destructive and, in desperation, people often make disastrous choices, perhaps leading to unfulfilling relationships and apparent promiscuity. Carers should beware of imposing feelings of inappropriate guilt on the patient.

With the diagnosis of AIDS people may experience many losses:

● loss of control
● loss of dignity
● loss of body image
● loss of a future

and an anticipated loss of any and everything that is important to them. Rejection, isolation and guilt may compound the feeling that the person is useless, hence their self esteem is lost.

Fears may be expressed, fear of dying, of the process and of what happens after death. Coming to terms with death and dying is painful even for those who have lived a full life but it must be so much more difficult for the many young people with AIDS.

The need to maintain hope

Absence of hope equals hopelessness and this is something that care professionals and their patients should not accept. There is never 'nothing that can be done'.

A friend had a biopsy of a lump in her breast. The result took ten days to come through. During that time she had gone through the various scenarios in her mind from the worst to the best. She felt she worked through a lot of issues but was very strong about this: 'The one thing I could not tolerate was them saying there is nothing they could do; I could not survive without hope.'

The need for honesty

In any caring situation mutual trust is essential and patients need to know that those caring for them will not mislead them or be dishonest with them. The degree of openness and discussion relating to sensitive issues is dependent on knowing the patient and respecting his wishes. The choice as to what information is disclosed, and the things that are better left unsaid, should be guided by a knowledge of the patient's coping mechanism.

The need to raise difficult and painful issues

When the patient trusts his carer it will be easier for the patient to raise difficult and painful issues. However, it is essential to recognise that some people's coping mechanism is found in denial (see Chapter 7). The patient may well be aware of their situation with all its implications but the last thing they want is to talk about it.

A young man who was experiencing short term memory loss would often ask members of the care team, 'Do I have AIDS?' He would move from reality to denial and finally back to reality. In the end he said, 'Did you know I have AIDS? Isn't it terrible, I hate it.'

He needed honesty coupled with reassurance that his worst fear of dying alone would not become a reality.

The need to overcome feelings of isolation

As mentioned at the beginning of this section, patients need freedom from isolation, rejection, guilt and fear. The isolation felt by people with

AIDS is probably something that few others have experienced to the same degree.

Peter, a patient with AIDS said, 'As a person with AIDS I feel isolated when I am with well people'.

A female patient said that when she was told of her HIV status, the most pressing need for her was to meet other women who were HIV Ab positive. Despite being surrounded by caring staff she felt alone in her pain and misery.

Not only do patients need reassurance that they will die comfortably and with dignity, with their wishes respected through dying and death, but also that they will not be alone.

The need for encouragement and motivation

In providing encouragement and motivation to help the person with AIDS get on with the business of living the personality of the carer is of great importance. There are patients who will do anything for a particular nurse and other nurses will just not achieve the same results. The carer must be flexible in his or her approach and remember that it is what the patient wants and needs that matters.

The need to be valued and to be of value

Every person cared for is of value and contributes much that is of great significance. The following was stated by Maria Swafford, a nurse working with AIDS programme in San Francisco:

We enter the lives of our patients at a very special but traumatic time – when they are confronting their imminent mortality. Often bonds of profound intimacy are forged through these trying circumstances and in the midst of tragedy care givers can facilitate opportunities for incredible emotional and spiritual growth by their patients and their families.

The need for the carer's time

Time spent performing tasks, listening or just time to be there are all important. Even when patients appear to be unconscious perhaps by just being there and holding a hand they can be reassured that they are not alone and given a sense of being cared for and about.

In order to respond to patients' emotional needs carers, whether statutory or voluntary, must have the following skills:

- The ability to listen and respond and also to know when to be silent.
- The ability to be able to find out where the patient 'is' regarding his situation, i.e. what he has been told and what he feels about it. It is important not to respond blindly to questions but rather build on what is known and work with the patient at his pace and in his time.
- The ability to recognise when it is necessary to refer to someone with greater skill; for example do not adopt the role of a trained and experienced counsellor unless qualified to do so.
- Carers must ensure that confidentiality is maintained; sharing something that has been told in confidence must only be done with the patient's permission.
- The ability to be able to love and accept people as they are. Attitudes toward people show in non-verbal communication long before any word is spoken. Sincerity and a genuine desire to care will be recognised; insincerity may be difficult to tolerate.

A young man with AIDS asked why so many people who met him for the first time felt it necessary to hug and kiss him. 'Is it this touch thing gone mad?' he said.

A young girl patient said that she had terrible stomach ache. 'If you stopped stuffing yourself full of cream toffees and Pepsi Cola you might feel better,' I replied. She stared at me for a minute, then laughed and said, 'Yeah'. We were always straight with each other and it made the relationship real.

As with all relationships it is not necessary for carers to agree with all aspects of the patient's life to love and accept them. Responding to a patient's emotional needs and helping them to deal with unfinished business will often be the release they needed and give them the freedom to get on with living.

Social needs

In responding to the social needs of people with AIDS it is important to liaise with social workers involved with the patient to identify the history and the current situation. Patients may have been involved with a social worker for some time and it is vital that, whenever possible, these links are maintained.

Housing and accommodation

The lack of suitable housing is a very big problem for the person with AIDS who:

● is homeless (they may have been homeless prior to becoming ill or have been evicted or asked to leave their accommodation for a variety of reasons including their diagnosis, their lifestyle, their colour, inability to pay rent, or arrears with mortgage payments)
● is unable to live alone
● lives alone but needs help
● can no longer climb flights of stairs and needs ground floor accommodation
● has become terminally ill and decides to sell his property or move from rented accommodation but then recovers
● is a mother caring for a baby in bed-sit accommodation.

It is often difficult to find accommodation for homeless people and there is no quick and easy way to solve this problem. Homeless people with a diagnosis of AIDS should be dealt with immediately wherever they are.

When caring for people with AIDS it is important to find out what the situation is regarding housing in their area and having done so to establish personal links with key personnel. In some areas housing associations are coming forward and expressing a willingness to house people with AIDS, either within general provision or in designated units. In Edinburgh the statutory services are selecting, training, and funding families who take people with AIDS into their homes. Training programmes for home helps can provide carers who are confident, and assistance that is both flexible and appropriate.

Hospitals with patients with AIDS should be flexible and allow well babies and toddlers to stay with their sick mothers. Assistance may be bought in from agencies for nursery nurses to be available for the period of the stay. Those involved in planning care should give thought to enabling families to stay together when the parents need care.

There are several organisations in the UK that may be able to give small grants to patients to assist with housing. These include the AIDS Care Education Trust (ACET), the Terrence Higgins Trust, Mainliners, and Body Positive. (See Appendix 1.)

In major cities the cost of accommodation for families and friends who may wish to visit a patient can be prohibitive. It is desirable for centres caring for people with AIDS to offer the opportunity for family or friends to stay overnight in the patient's room and/or to provide accommodation (e.g. an apartment or room) within the centre.

24-hour care

Is home care really an option for those people with AIDS who are living alone and need 24-hour nursing care or 24-hour supervisory care?

For those living alone and housebound a considerable amount of assistance with shopping, cleaning and food preparation may be needed from home helps and/or volunteers. A mother with AIDS may need help in caring for her baby – at the moment this help is usually given by friends, or relatives.

Finance

People with AIDS need to know the allowances that may be available to them and how to gain access to these allowances. Benefits from Social Services and grants from charitable agencies may include:

- Housing Benefit
- Disabled Living Allowance
- Disabled Working Allowance
- Social fund – crisis loans
- Sickness Benefit
- Income Support
- Invalidity Benefit (after 28 weeks).

Further information may be sought from the Department of Social Services, ACET and THT. See also Appendixes 1 and 2.

Many patients may also have fears and anxieties for the future of their partner and family, especially if they have been the main provider of income or they are a single parent. Carers should be able to reassure the patient and to advise on the benefits and income support systems available.

It is important to recognise when a patient may need financial help, not only to provide for their own (and their families') everyday needs such as food and accommodation, but to help in maintaining their quality of life. For example, most people with AIDS will have lost a considerable amount of weight and be demoralised by having to appear in ill-fitting clothes which emphasise the altered body image – the ability to be able to purchase new clothes may have a very positive effect on their morale. Patients may also gain pleasure from being able to afford to buy a small present for their carer(s) or a member of their family.

People with AIDS may be sharing mortgages or rents with their partner or family member and may need advice and assistance in sorting out the legal and financial issues involved.

Spiritual needs

When people are ill and activity is restricted they will often, for the first time in many busy years, have time to reflect about the meaning and purpose of their life. This may be a painful process and involve them in examining areas of guilt and conflict as well as contemplating their value and belief systems. Many will need help and support from their carers during this time (see also Chapter 8). Given a safe, secure, loving environment free from pressure, ridicule and judgemental attitudes, people will feel more able to explore and express their spiritual needs, conflicts and problems. People's religious beliefs, or the fact that they have no religious belief, must be respected.

Carers must recognise that

- patients need to have the freedom to worship according to their faith and this should be facilitated whenever possible
- some patients will need to have the sacraments brought to them, others will derive great comfort by being taken to a place of worship
- the need for pastoral care may be met by the hospital chaplain or by another spiritual advisor of the patient's own choosing
- the patient may need to discuss issues relating to his funeral service.

Patients must not be pressurised regarding their spiritual needs, but it is important not to neglect this area of care. Patients may experience a need for forgiveness of themselves, of others, and a sense of being forgiven by God and/or others before they can find peace of mind.

Until people with AIDS know that they can trust the carer, and that acceptance of them and friendship to them is genuine, the carer will not be in a position to share with them issues relating to their most fundamental needs.

Reference

Wilkes, E., Harnett, G., Speed, D. *et al.* (1980). *Report of the Working Group on Terminal Care.* HMSO, London.

3

The multiprofessional team

'So in everything, do to others what you would have them do to you'

Matthew 7:12

When the declared aims of care are to provide for the needs of the whole person it is not always possible, or even good, for one person to provide all the care. One person does not usually have the expertise or the time that is needed. It would also encourage too great a dependence on one person; when that particular carer is unavailable or fails in some way, it is possible that the whole care package can fall apart. At their best, multiprofessional teams can ensure that all the needs of the patient are met. The team must have a common approach and understanding of the overall aim, but team members must also have an understanding of, and respect for, each other's expertise. Good communication regarding each profession's codes of conduct and policies, as well as about subjects directly related to the care of a particular person, enables the team to work together with mutual respect and understanding. This can be achieved through regular multiprofessional team meetings, at case conferences where appropriate, as well as through the use of the telephone or in direct discussion with the appropriate team member.

Aims of care

Each individual team member will have their own philosophy or belief systems which will affect how the care is delivered. Each discipline also has its own code of practice but to achieve a coordinated approach it is important that the team as a whole agrees on the overall aims of care. The aims should include the following:

- To provide for the needs of the whole person.
- To treat each person as an individual, with respect and acceptance, acknowledging each person's right to privacy and confidentiality.

- To give control back to the patient as far as is possible.
- To enhance the quality of life by good care, including aids for daily living, appropriate housing and effective symptom control, enabling the patient to live life as fully as possible until death.
- To facilitate a comfortable and dignified death.
- To provide support and bereavement follow up to families, partners and friends, recognising all who are of importance to the patient.

The multiprofessional team

Ideally, the core of the team should include nurses, a doctor, therapists, a dietitian, social workers, counsellors and psychologists, and chaplains and ministers of religion, either to give regular input or to be available when needed or wanted.

Nurses

The nurses, together with the partner or family of the patient, provide the greatest input to care of the terminally ill person with AIDS. Professor Eric Wilkes in his report on the working party on terminal care in 1980 commented, rightly, that good terminal care depends, in the main, on good nursing (Wilkes et al., 1980). Nurses are privileged to provide the most intimate details of care, and are also the first to whom the patients will turn for advice or for a listening ear. Nurses are also in a good position to observe and monitor symptoms and developing problems, as well as the response to symptom control management and medication. In the community in Britain, the district nursing services have for many years worked with the primary nursing model, ideally with the primary nurse as the coordinator of the care given to any one patient. Good communication between the nurses and doctors is of the greatest importance in order to achieve good symptom control and medical management. Nursing issues are dealt with in Chapter 4.

Doctors

The doctor's role and medical issues are dealt with in more detail in Chapters 5 and 6, but suffice it to say here that the doctor is but one member of the team and should communicate closely with other members of the team, in particular with the nurses. The doctor's most obvious roles here are in symptom control and the management of medical problems directly related to AIDS. However, the doctor should also be available to the team for advice and discussion in order to contribute to the whole, as well as being available to each individual patient and his family to give information, advice, and support. When the patient dies the doctor has practical matters to deal with, such as death certificates and cremation forms, but he should also be available for on-going support to the family who may have questions and worries that need to be dealt with.

Therapists

Physiotherapists have an important role to play in maintaining quality of life for as long as possible, in easing or comforting distressing muscle aches and pains, and in relieving some of the breathing difficulties related to chest infections. They may also have a great deal to contribute to such problems as seating, lifting, and those related to the chronic disabilities that often occur with the slowly progressive neurological forms of the disease. Some patients who appear to be moribund may recover and then require rehabilitation with very active physiotherapy input.

Occupational therapists also have an important role, and, in liaison with physiotherapists, may help to achieve a great improvement in the quality of life through improving functions and activities of daily living, enabling the patient to maintain independence for as long as possible.

Input from therapists can be invaluable in the community, enabling the patient to live at home through the use of adaptations or aids that are available for daily living. Other therapies should also be available according to the needs and wishes of the individual patient; for example art therapy may not only provide stimulation to creativity, and occupation, but may also enable the patient to express feelings and emotions that he is unable to talk about.

Dietitian

Dietetic advice is, of course, an important aspect of the overall care for the person with AIDS. As the illness progresses eating difficulties may increase. Some patients may experiment with a variety of diets, hoping to combat the disease and its progress. Some diets undoubtedly contribute to the development of malnutrition, particularly in those who already have persistent and severe diarrhoea, as occurs in cryptosporidiosis. As the illness progresses and becomes more debilitating problems of nausea, dysphagia or intractable vomiting may develop and total parenteral nutrition (TPN) may be instituted. It is quite possible to maintain TPN in the community, but good liaison is essential between the dietitian, the doctors, the pharmacists and the laboratory involved. In these cases difficult decisions as to how long TPN should be continued in the terminal care setting will need to be faced (see also Chapters 5 and 6).

Social workers

Many of the social needs of patients with AIDS have been discussed in Chapter 2. As the illness progresses, and as patients become more debilitated or disabled by neurological problems such as caused by HIV encephalopathy, cerebral toxoplasmosis and progressive multifocal leucoencephalopathy (PML) (see Chapter 6), housing, financial and general support and supervision needs may become more and more difficult to deal with. Single parents who have small children may worry about their children being taken into care, or about what will happen to their children when they die. Financial problems may be weighing very heavily and will require sensitive handling. The complexities of welfare benefit, legal problems, funeral expenses and the making of wills may all seem very daunting; sorting these out may make a very big difference to the quality of those last few weeks or months of life. Psychiatric social workers may be involved together with psychiatrists in sorting out problems that have arisen as a result of developing HIV encephalopathy, such as the disinhibited, sometimes manic behaviours that may be an early sign of dementia even in the late stages of the syndrome. In some hospitals and hospices, and sometimes in the community, social workers may be involved in counselling, in liaison with psychologists and psychiatrists. There may be serious family conflict over wills in which the social workers or counsellors may find themselves having to take on the role of mediators (see also Chapters 2 and 7).

Counsellors and psychologists

Strong counselling input will be needed, both to the patient and to those close to him, to provide support during the patient's illness and also bereavement follow-up and counselling as necessary after death. Counsellors and welfare assistants need to work very closely together, as some of the counselling input deals with the matters discussed in the above section on social work. However many issues relate to death and dying, to family conflicts, and to relationships which are often very complex, such as an ex-spouse and children visiting a patient whose present partner is also visiting and between whom there might be considerable antagonism. Parents, particularly fathers, have often not been able to accept their son's gay relationship. (Many of these issues are looked at in more detail in Chapter 7.) The work of the counsellor or psychologist will often overlap into spiritual or pastoral care as patients express deep conflict, doubts, anger, guilt and fear. It is important that counsellors and psychologists recognise the contribution that the chaplain or ministers of religion have to make in this area, and that each respects the other and works together with the patient to achieve peace of mind.

Chaplains and ministers of religion

Spiritual and pastoral care issues are dealt with in Chapter 8. These should be seen as having an important contribution to make to the whole care of the person who is living with AIDS, particularly as he enters the terminal phases. This is the time when the person needs strong reassurance, understanding, empathy, simple friendship and access to those important sacraments or rituals that reinforce a sense of belonging and of confidence. Uncomplicated and unconditional acceptance and love, creating a sense of security and of trust between the patient and his spiritual adviser, will enable the patient to explore doubts, fears, beliefs or non beliefs without fear of ridicule or rejection. However, the barriers will remain firmly up if he senses condemnation, judgement or even fear of the illness itself on the part of the chaplain.

A team which communicates and is well coordinated has the potential for providing very high standards of care. However, with such a number of people involved the potential for confusion is also great. The patient may not be able to, or wish to, relate to so many people and may prefer to communicate deeply with only one or two members of the team, or may find his support elsewhere. Someone who has recently become blind, or who is severely debilitated and ill, may become totally confused and withdrawn if he is being forced to relate to too many people. In this situation it is important that the team agrees amongst itself who is the best person to be the key worker. This is likely to be the primary nurse but it could be anyone with whom the patient communicates well. It is important also that issues of confidentiality are understood and respected within the team. The patient may not be at all happy about matters that he has discussed with one person being passed on to the rest of the team. Anyone who has been the recipient of sensitive or confidential information should always check with the patient first before divulging the details to other team members.

Categories of care

The continuum of care in advanced disease is non acute and different categories of care may be required. These categories include:

- respite care
- rehabilitative or convalescent care
- terminal care

- bereavement support and follow up (this is most commonly offered in the home or in a hospice).

Respite care

For patients being cared for at home, particularly those who are severely debilitated or disabled, respite care may provide a much needed and sometime essential change, not only for the patient but also for the carer. For the patient respite care may provide an opportunity for time and space on their own, but with all the necessities of life being provided by a professional team in the comfort of a hospice or nursing home. For the carers it may provide a break from the exhaustion of continually caring for someone close to them. Regular respite admissions every six to eight weeks may enable patients to remain at home through most of their illness, particularly if this is taking a slowly progressive form. Respite may also be provided on a day basis once or twice a week at a day centre. In admitting patients for respite care it may become apparent that the patient is terminally ill and in need of more intensive nursing care and support than that which is possible to provide in the community. Admission may then need to be arranged in response to a crisis situation.

Convalescent and rehabilitative care

Patients requiring convalescence or rehabilitation will be recovering from an acute illness or an apparent terminal phase (patients referred for terminal care may recover and require rehabilitative care). Physiotherapy and occupational therapy input is particularly important in this group of patients. Physiotherapy may also be of value in the day care or home setting for patients who have had neurological problems.

All these categories of care provision will be increasingly necessary during the next five years, even in the unlikely event of a cure or vaccine being found within the next few years. Patients requiring long term care or continuing care – people who are seriously debilitated or disabled by the virus, people who may have permanent neurological problems such as HIV related encephalopathy, hemiplegias or severe neuropathy – will present particular problems in the community.

Sheltered or supervised accommodation, or accommodation adapted for disabled people is already desperately needed, especially in the larger cities. Continuing input will be required from all health care professionals, with intensification of input from time to time, particularly as people become terminally ill.

Patient-directed care and the multiprofessional team

Good team work may result in excellent provision of care. However, it must always be remembered that the patient is the hub of the wheel and should, as far as possible, be in control at all times. There is also, as has been mentioned, the potential for confusion, manipulation and misunderstanding particularly if communication breaks down between team members and the patient, or the patient plays one team member off against the other.

A patient in our care appeared to be very confused, and also had all of us confused. We eventually found out that there had been more than 20 people or agencies involved in his care in the community, most of whom did not know of the others' existence until a meeting was set up to which the patient was also invited. The patient appeared to be in control, but was in fact suffering from the early effects of HIV encephalopathy.

Patient-directed care in practice and at its best means that the patient is in control, working with the different members of the multiprofessional team who inform, advise and enable him to make valid choices out of the available options. The options available will vary from time to time and the patient's ability to make choices will also vary according to his health, both physical and emotional. Many professionals, particularly doctors and perhaps nurses, are used to being directive in their approach to patients. At times the patient prefers or needs directive care and skill is required to know when this is appropriate. Sometimes the patient makes it clear that this is what he wants and then his wish should, of course, be respected, unless the patient is abdicating all responsibility, thereby increasing his dependency and illness.

A patient admitted for rehabilitation was very demotivated and unwilling to cooperate with any attempts at rehabilitation. At first his need to be left alone and to abdicate responsibility was accepted and respected; however, it became clear that this attitude was seriously affecting his progress and health – he was not terminally ill. He was challenged from time to time by different members of the team to take up that responsibility again for himself. A consistent approach had to be developed by the team and he was eventually able to take up the responsibility, take part in the case conference and discharge planning, and eventually to go home.

In practice, patient-directed care means that ward routine has to be flexible, sometimes with a considerable amount of negotiation between patient, nurse and other patients to ensure harmonious communal living. It may mean that times for visits from physiotherapists or counsellors may have to be negotiated with the patient to fit in with other plans that he may have. It means that the patient is given whatever information he needs or wants in order to be able to make informed choices. This includes information regarding medication – some patients know a great deal about the different medications that they are taking, particularly those related to AIDS, for example zidovudine. Patients with AIDS will often be very informed about the latest research into new drugs, for example drugs that are available in America but not in the UK, and herbal or other remedies which are being tried in various countries. Doctors and nurses in particular need to keep themselves well informed in order to be able to discuss the pros and cons of a particular medication or regime.

Inherent in this approach to care is a risk that the advice given may be rejected, the care or even the carer may not be wanted or appreciated. This can be particularly difficult for care givers to accept or understand. Professional carers are used to patients being grateful, passive and cooperative. Patients who are not, are quickly labelled difficult, or sometimes even psychotic.

A patient who refused a number of investigations and treatments that were being advised and who had been travelling to and from hospital frequently and felt himself to be deteriorating, refused to accept any further active intervention. He felt that he was being pressurised, by the doctors, against his will, became very angry when he was referred to a psychiatrist and walked out. His partner was told that he had become psychotic and needed psychiatric intervention and possibly admission to a psychiatric unit. His partner eventually found him wandering around the streets of London in a very exhausted state, brought him home and persuaded him to come to Mildmay for some respite on the understanding that he would not be forced into anything that he did not wish to have done.

For the first few days he was extremely suspicious, very withdrawn and refused all nursing and medical care including any medication. If asked if he wanted a drink or food he would say no. He was in total body pain and had severe oral thrush, which made his mouth sore and swallowing difficult. The doctor, on introducing herself was asked why she thought she knew what was best for him and was told to get out. Nurses were told that they were not wanted, he only wanted to be left alone. It was clear that he was very angry and suspicious, and he needed time and space to himself in order to build up some trust in what we had to offer.

The nurses and the doctor continued to go in from time to time to explain briefly that he did not need to continue in pain and that his mouth could be made much more comfortable with some nystatin suspension. When cups of tea were brought in and left for him to drink, he sometimes drank them. He slowly began to trust that he would not be forced into any action to which he did not agree and built up a rapport with one of the nurses through whom he finally agreed to have 4 hourly morphine for his pain and nystatin for his oral thrush.

As he began to feel more comfortable he began to lose his suspicion and distrust. His partner was able to spend much time with him. Eventually the patient was able to make informed choices about his care, deal with a number of matters which, for him, were matters of unfinished business, renew and deepen relationships with the family. He died with a sense of achievement and at peace within himself. The end result was very rewarding for all concerned but the process involved a considerable amount of risk, and many painful encounters for staff.

Some patients are very skilled at manipulation; maybe they have had to spend most of their lives fighting to achieve good, or in 'beating the system'. Some patients' personalities are altered by HIV encephalopathy and some people are just manipulative. In such situations it is important that the team communicates, has a common approach which all members of the team understand and apply consistently, and that the boundaries are firmly and clearly explained to the patient. Freedom within boundaries can give a great sense of security and can still enable the patient to feel in control or to take responsibility. The boundaries and freedoms may require a certain amount of negotiation, but once agreed they should be seen as a contract that is binding to both parties, and treated as such. Again it is important that the contract is understood not only by the patient but by every member of the team.

This approach to care can be costly to staff who are used to a more directive or authoritarian approach, but it can also be immensely rewarding. In giving control back to the patient and placing responsibility where it belongs, with him, it can often also give him back a sense of identity and of worth, together with a restoration of his will to live.

A patient, having lived for several weeks with considerable quality of life, said ten days before he died, 'The people here gave me back my will to live; this is the greatest gift that anyone can give to another human being'.

Reference

Wilkes, E., Harnett, G., Speed, D. *et al.* (1980). *Report of the Working Group on Terminal Care.* HMSO, London.

4

Nursing issues

'The unique function of the nurse is to assist the individual, sick or well, in the performance of those activities, contributing to health or its recovery (or to a peaceful death) that he would perform unaided, if he had the necessary strength, will and knowledge.'

Henderson (1958)

The Wilkes (1980) report described terminal care as 'the provision of the very special support required by (terminally ill) patients and their families, and it is based, above all, on high quality nursing'.

Many people with AIDS are reminded of the reality of their situation every time they look into the mirror and see their wasted body or disfiguring lesions. To encourage these people to see value in life and carry on living takes considerable skill. Nurses need to utilise all their skills and ensure that their knowledge is adequately maintained in this developing area of care.

People with AIDS are often young people, facing a terminal illness, and many the same age as the nurses who are caring for them. These people may

- be emerging from the control of parents and/or educational and training establishments into a situation where they control and manage their lives, perhaps for the first time
- be living chaotic life styles, 'no one telling them what to do'
- as adults, have just found answers to conflicts affecting their lives, and have started 'really living' for the first time
- have worked hard and moved up the promotional ladder to positions of responsibility or set up their own businesses, and are now at the peak of their career with 'the world as their oyster'.

Faced at this time, therefore, with the loss of the future they had hoped and planned for, it is not surprising that the majority of people with AIDS need to retain control over their lives.

The environment of care

People's homes vary enormously, but wherever they are and whatever they are like they usually offer security and safety. In their own home the occupant feels a sense of belonging, surrounded by 'their' things, things that are important to them and with which they are familiar. In their own home people can invite some in, keep others out, and be alone when they need to; they can eat, drink, wash, work and sleep when they choose to. People who do not live alone may not have the same ability to control their environment but will usually have a situation of negotiation and 'give and take'.

When care is given in a hospital or hospice *the environment should be made as comfortable and as home-like as possible.* Patients who are likely to be in hospital or hospice for any length of time should be encouraged to bring in some small items from home, items that are important to him. The availability of books, magazines and tapes will help in providing a comfortable environment, as will an amenity fund from which flowers and extras can be bought for patients who have very little.

If patients are to have single rooms (consumer research at Mildmay indicates that this is clearly their preference) it is important that there are communal facilities where they can be with other people when they so wish. The privacy of their rooms should be respected and the patient consulted before visitors are allowed. It may be necessary to use 'please do not disturb' labels on doors to ensure that patients who need to rest are not disturbed by any of the team members without first consulting the nurse caring for that patient.

When a patient dies it is often appropriate that they are viewed in their own rooms, where 'good byes' can be said in a room that speaks of its resident, with familiar objects that speak of the living that took place in the midst of dying.

Flexibility

It is possible for patients to retain control over their lives whether they are being cared for in hospital, at home or in a hospice. In order to give patients control it is necessary for nurses to be given a greater degree of freedom and flexibility within the structure in which they work, so as not to be bound by routine and rigid time-tables. It will be necessary to ensure that managers understand the philosophy for nursing care so that inflexibility on their part does not restrict practice.

The structure in which care professionals work, the environment and inadequate resources may hinder the giving of control to patients. Lack of finance hinders every aspect of provision.

If there is only one bath, one shower, does this render routine essential?

Is service provision geared to patient needs or does the patient have to fit in with the system?

Dare you, can you change things in an established routine?

With the resistance of many carers to any change, and the directive attitude of many doctors and therapists, can you change to what may be a very different way of working?

What will help the nurse to make these changes?

- Acceptance of the need of most patients, not just those with AIDS, to have control.
- Confidence in the nurse's own ability to cope with the outcomes of giving control to patients.
- The need and the opportunity for nurses to examine and evaluate their practice.

The routine that involves learners in washing and getting up Mrs Smith, Mrs Brown and Mrs Jones before they go to coffee is still evident in some training hospitals. It is still possible to visit wards where the rules for nurses are 'Thou shalt not eat and drink on the ward'. What about when the best way to encourage a patient to eat is to take a meal with him? The hospitals and hospices which demonstrate flexibility and give control to patients are places where patients are living and positive attitudes are in evidence.

Relationships between the nurse, the patient and those close to him

Relationships with all patients should be based on mutual trust and acceptance and be confident and relaxed. Ensuring that one's knowledge and skills are adequate will enhance self confidence in the nurse, which in turn will inspire confidence in the patient and those close to him.

Primary nursing facilitates the establishment of good relationships between nurses and their patients and ensures continuity of care. It also allows nursing staff greater autonomy. Each patient has a specific nurse, or nurses, with whom they can identify and work in partnership, so creating an environment suitable for making choices (Ersser and Tutton, 1990).

Rejection

Nurses usually find themselves in a situation of being needed and liked by their patients. This varies, of course, according to their area of care but most nurses enjoy the sharing in people's lives that nursing involves. The unresolved understandable anger that a few people with AIDS may have, at times presents itself in the need to reject others, including the nurse.

A patient said to one nurse, 'If you think I find talking therapeutic, then you're wrong', and turned away every time she appeared. The nurse did not find the patient as hard to handle as her own feelings of being rejected, especially when talking was therapeutic for the patient with other nurses.

Some patients have not liked male nurses, female nurses or one nurse in particular. This problem is particularly apparent with patients with AIDS, perhaps because such patients feel that they are more able to make their own choices.

In dealing with rejection it is essential that nurses try to understand why the patient behaves in this way. It is important not to make assumptions but to establish facts. Nurses may need help and support (often from peers) to enable them to accept that the rejection is usually not personal but rejection of the system or displaced anger. If it is personal, the nurse needs to determine why someone responds to them in that way and, if possible, to remedy the situation. The nurse may need help and advice to see how he is perceived by others. Working together as a team and talking through difficulties with colleagues is often extremely helpful. In most instances the problems will be resolved, not by allowing the patient to make unreasonable demands, but by facing up to difficult problems with the patient and challenging when necessary. Giving patients choices may result in a patient refusing care from a particular nurse, and will present nurses with problems – problems that they must work through in order to be able to fulfil the duty of care they have to all patients.

Fear

Many nurses may be apprehensive about caring for people who are HIV antibody positive. Often it is not so much fear that they will become infected themselves, but that they might take 'something' home to their families and/or loved ones. The nurse's family may put pressure on the nurse, making it clear that they are not happy that he or she should expose him or herself, or them, to risk. These attitudes show that, although efforts have been made to educate and reassure, doubt, fear and misconception still exist. Television and newspaper reports often provide conflicting evidence, giving cause for concern. It is possible that, for many nurses, it is just 'fear of the unknown' that worries them, especially those nurses who have not yet cared for people with AIDS.

Relationships within the multiprofessional team

Whilst nurses have a key role in the terminal care of people with AIDS it is important that, by being 'jack of all trades', they do not exclude experts from other disciplines. It is often appropriate that the clinical nurse in charge is the coordinator of the multiprofessional team as she will be likely to have in-depth information on all the patients (see also Chapter 3).

Principles of nursing care

In any care setting the principles of nursing care will be the same (see also Chapter 2).

- The unit of care is the patient and those important to him, be they family, partners or friends.
- Total nursing care is given to each patient as an appropriate response to their individual needs.
- The practice of nursing ensures continuity of care for the patient – this may involve visiting the patient prior to admission. Visits from community staff prior to discharge should be encouraged.
- Nurses encourage care to be self-directed by patients whenever possible. It may be necessary with some patients to provide a framework, agreed boundaries, within which a patient has control.
- The nurse works in partnership with the patient toward the achievement of his aims and goals. The setting of short term achievable goals is a good motivating force.
- The emphasis should be on enhancing quality of life. It is important to make the most of every day and to make each day special.

Giving control where it belongs – to the patients – is often easier said than done. It involves

- accepting a challenge
- having the courage to change things
- being innovative – working out new ways of solving problems
- being willing to accept difficult outcomes
- taking risks.

But above all it involves reinforcing the value that carers place on those they care for.

Infection control

If the care of people with AIDS is the nurses' responsibility, how are they going to deliver effective care to the patient while minimising the risk of infection to themselves and other patients? The US Centers for Disease Control Surveillance studies show that the risk of acquiring HIV from a single needlestick injury involving blood from an HIV infected person is LESS than 0.5%. The risk of hepatitis B transmission from high risk patients from a similar injury is 20%.

Transmission of the virus may occur sexually, perinatally, by inoculation, *in utero*, and via breast milk. No other routes of spread are known. Therefore, the most important infection control measures are based on the prevention of inoculation accidents with used 'sharps', and the avoidance of frank contamination of skin and mucous membranes with blood and other body fluids.

The following body fluids should be handled with the same precautions as blood:

- cerebrospinal fluid
- peritoneal fluid
- pleural fluid
- synovial fluid
- amniotic fluid
- semen
- vaginal secretions
- any other body fluid containing visible blood
- saliva in association with dentistry
- unfixed tissues and organs.

Gloves should be used to protect the health care worker in the following situations (the type of glove used – surgical, examination or household – will depend on the task):

- all procedures in all patients where contamination of the health care workers with blood is probable
- venepuncture when:
    - the venepuncturist is inexperienced
    - the patient is restless
    - the patient is known to be infected with HIV or bloodborne hepatitis virus
- when cleaning equipment prior to sterilisation or disinfection
- when handling chemical disinfectants
- when cleaning up spillages of blood.

Table 1. Task categorisation according to risk of exposure to blood (HMSO 1990)

	Category	Examples	Protective measures
A(i)	Contact of health care worker with blood probable; potential for uncontrolled bleeding or spattering	Major surgical, gynaecological and obstetrical procedures	Full range of protective clothing
A(ii)	Contact of health care worker with blood probable but spattering unlikely	Intra-arterial punctures. Insertion/removal of intravenous/intra-arterial lines	Gloves to be worn. Masks/ protective eyewear to be available
A(iii)	Low probability of personal contact	Administration of intramuscular, intradermal or subcutaneous injections	Gloves available

Ways to avoid exposure to HIV and bloodborne hepatitis viruses in the health care setting

- Apply good basic hygiene practices with regular hand washing.
- Cover existing wounds or skin lesions with waterproof dressings.
- Take simple protective measures to avoid contamination of person and clothing with blood.
- Protect mucous membrane of eyes, mouth and nose from blood splashes.
- Prevent puncture wounds, cuts and abrasions in the presence of blood.
- Avoid sharps usage wherever possible.
- Institute a safe procedure for handling and disposal of sharps.
- Clear up spillages of blood promptly and disinfect surfaces.
- Institute a procedure for the safe disposal of contaminated waste.

Members of staff who are immunodeficient/compromised either through illness or therapy, or suffering from exfoliative skin conditions should seek the advice of the occupational health department before nursing patients who are HIV positive.

The nurse must be aware of procedures which exist for the management of equipment, waste and linen which are potentially contaminated with opportunistic infective organisms. There may be local variations but there are certain general points. In the National Health Service in the UK, disposable contaminated articles and rubbish are placed in heavy duty yellow plastic bags, no other labelling being required. It is essential that needles and sharp ends of tubing should be removed and placed in a 'sharps' bin and not in the plastic bag. The yellow bags and 'sharps' bins are then incinerated. Linen soiled with blood and body fluids should be double bagged in red bags. The inner bag will be water soluble plastic and the outer red nylon. The red bags will be recognised as containing infected linen and no other labelling is required. In some areas a service is provided to patients in the community which involves the collection of infected, and the distribution of clean, linen.

Local policy will determine whether the nurse has a responsibility to decontaminate autoclavable and non-autoclavable instruments and equipment prior to return to CSSD. It will also determine how this is to be performed. Although HIV can be inactivated by most disinfectants, since people with AIDS frequently have several opportunistic infections, disinfectants which are mycobacteriocidal, for example glutaraldehyde, are used for disinfecting all instruments which cannot be autoclaved. If not otherwise specified, used instruments should be bagged and labelled according to local policy and returned to CSSD. All rubbish not contaminated with blood and body fluids should be placed in the black plastic bags (non-infected waste) (see also p.152).

Home care

In many areas local authorities arrange for collection of waste for incineration and, as already stated, a few also have laundry services for infected linen.

Protective clothing in the form of plastic aprons and gloves should be available for staff and family/friends who assist with personal care, and the nurse should ensure that carers know when and when not to use them, and why.

Bins for sharps, and disinfectants (household bleach diluted 1:10 with water) and/or Presept granules or tablets should be kept in the house.

The household crockery and cutlery may be used by the patient; it is not necessary to keep separate utensils. Soiled linen can be washed satisfactorily on the hot cycle of a domestic washing machine. People with HIV can use the same toilet, bath and shower as the rest of the household and it will not need disinfecting after use.

It is NOT necessary to wear protective clothing of any sort for normal social contact with the patient, such as delivering food, post, counselling, chatting, pushing a wheelchair, shaking a patient's hand, or even giving him/her a hug.

In summary, the only precautions necessary (unless specifically stated) will be the use of gloves and aprons by those carers handling blood and body fluids. The same rule applies whether the patient is being cared for in hospital, in the community, or in a hospice.

The educational needs of nurses

In order to provide effective care nurses will need a comprehensive induction programme and on-going education and training to ensure a knowledge and understanding of related issues including

- the stigma of AIDS
- issues relating to altered body image and death and dying
- symptom control for people with AIDS
- listening and counselling skills
- issues relating to sexuality and drug addiction.

Support for nurses

It is recognised that nurses working in terminal care need considerable support, especially when coping with multiple bereavements. Wherever possible it is important that the structure within which they work is supportive in terms of the following:

- manpower – adequate staffing levels with an appropriate skill mix
- environment – absence of unnecessary rules and regulations
- resources – adequate equipment to assist in giving high quality care
- provision of appropriate training
- commitment to staff development
- availability and interest of the manager.

In order to provide emotional support for staff in any setting it is essential to identify what it is that staff find to be helpful. Some nurses may find it helpful to talk to a counsellor on a one to one basis, others may find support groups of more value. Many will find their support by sharing with their peers, the friends they have made in their work setting. It is important not to overdo 'support', resulting in staff who find they are suddenly overwhelmed with problems they didn't even know they had.

The comment made by Richard Wells in the foreword of Pratt (1989) provides a fitting conclusion to this chapter.

The lack of a biomedical response to AIDS offers nursing the opportunity – probably for the first time – to prove what nursing is worth and to demonstrate that although the eventual outcome cannot be changed, the path to the outcome can be made less rigorous and more tolerable through nursing's interventions.

References

Ersser, S. and Tutton, E. (Eds) (1990). *Primary Nursing in Perspective.* Scutari Press, London.

Henderson, V. (1958). *Basis Principles of Nursing Care.* International Council of Nurses, London.

HMSO (1990). *Guidance for Clinical Health Care Workers: Protection against HIV and Hepatitis Viruses.* HMSO, London.

Pratt, R. (1989). *AIDS: a Strategy for Nursing Care,* second edition. Edward Arnold, London.

Wilkes, E., Harnett, G., Speed, D. *et al.* (1980). *Report of the Working Group on Terminal Care.* HMSO, London.

5

Medical issues and dilemmas

Robert was a highly respected and much travelled business man in his 50s. When admitted to Mildmay for terminal care he was intermittently confused, very non-communicative, doubly incontinent, required 2-hourly turning, and refused to take food and drink for most of the time. His skin was very dry, he had seborrhoeic dermatitis, most noticeably on his face, and lymphoedema of the left leg with a large Kaposi's sarcoma (KS) lesion on the shin and a smaller one on the dorsal aspect of the foot. He had hepatomegaly, oral candidosis and dysphagia. Four months previously Robert had presented at a hospital with a dark purplish spreading lesion on the left shin, and complaining of tiredness. He had also noticed that his memory was not as good as usual, but had put this down to pressure at work and tiredness. Robert had noticed the lesion on his shin and one or two other smaller lesions elsewhere for several months beforehand but had not sought medical advice. He had also had intermittent diarrhoea from time to time and had lost some weight.

The biopsy of one of the purplish lesions showed that this was due to Kaposi's sarcoma and he was found to be HIV antibody positive. Further investigations revealed atypical mycobacteria in his stool and bone marrow – this was, on culture, found to be *Mycobacterium avium intracellulare* (MAI). A CT scan showed that he had mild cerebral atrophy. His KS lesions were treated with radiotherapy and he was started on anti-tuberculous treatment. As Robert had a history of herpes simplex infections, and one year prior to his diagnosis had had an episode of herpes zoster, he was also given acyclovir prophylactically.

During the following three months Robert's condition deteriorated quickly. He continued to have problems with diarrhoea, vomiting and loss of weight. The KS lesions became more numerous and one in particular, on his left foot, caused swelling and discomfort in the foot with increased difficulty in walking. He became less and less mobile, increasingly depressed, more and more withdrawn and, at a later stage, intermittently confused. Robert gave his brother power of attorney.

When Robert was admitted to Mildmay, time was initially spent by the nursing team and the doctors in assessing his most obvious symptoms and dealing effectively with these. The nurses, in particular, spent time listening and just being with him and his partner. When he refused to take medication, this was discussed with him in detail by the doctor; his wishes to stop anti-TB medication and acyclovir were respected. However, with some negotiation he agreed to take those medications that had a direct effect on symptoms, including ketoconazole and nystatin oral suspension.

As his symptoms came under control, partly as a result of the care that he was receiving and partly as a result of stopping his anti-TB medication which had been contributing considerably to his nausea, Robert began to eat and drink small quantities again. As he regained a sense of control he also regained an interest in life, became less withdrawn and confused. Ten days after admission he took his first walk down to the lounge. During the following week he agreed to re-start his anti-TB medication and, as his improvement continued, he requested radiotherapy for the KS on his left foot.

Robert took back his power of attorney and started holding business meetings from his room, sorting out his personal and business affairs. He was able to go home again to live independently with his partner (with whom he had lived for many years) for a short while before he was finally re-admitted for terminal care. In his final admission Robert once again required total nursing care, his HIV encephalopathy having progressed so that his symptoms were once again out of control. These were quickly brought under control and Robert died comfortably and with dignity several months after his initial admission.

Robert's story illustrates a number of medical dilemmas that are familiar to anyone dealing with life-threatening illnesses. It also illustrates some issues which are directly related to AIDS. Direct symptom control details are dealt with in Chapter 6. This chapter considers some of the specific dilemmas and issues that are raised by the person with AIDS in the terminal care setting.

Is death synonymous with failure?

Doctors are generally trained to save life, or to prolong it, sometimes at great cost to the patient and to his carers. In an acute hospital setting death is often seen as a failure on the part of science and on the part of the doctors. The hospice movement has, in the past 20 years or so, taught us that death need not always be seen as a failure, or as an enemy. It may sometimes be a friend. When it is known, and accepted, that death is inevitable it is the quality of life that matters, not the quantity.

If Robert had died within the first week or two of his admission, perhaps his death could have been seen as a failure. With good symptom control and nursing care, and being given time, his interest in life was re-awakened. As he regained the sense of control he also regained his sense of identity and purpose. He was able to sort out his business affairs and leave his own personal affairs in good order. The quality of life for him and his partner included time together, first in the hospice unit and then at home.

As Robert's disease progressed, and in particular as the HIV encephalopathy became more obvious, his quality of life again changed for the worse. When re-admitted for terminal care he had had time to prepare himself and was now ready to face death. This time death was not a failure either by him or by the doctors, although it could be said to have been a failure of science in that a cure had not been found. However, an understanding of the principles of palliative medicine (a science in itself) had enabled the team to achieve comfort and dignity of the patient.

Prognosis and unpredictability

One of the most frequent questions a doctor is asked when dealing with a patient with a life threatening illness, is 'How long will it be, doctor? How long does he have?' This is always a difficult question to answer and the doctor who is foolhardy enough to give a definite statement will usually be proved wrong. This is particularly true for people with AIDS. AIDS is, as yet, a 'new' disease, with much to be learnt about the natural progress of the disease in its many different manifestations. The patients are often young, with a strong will to live and to remain in control, often persisting with active treatment until the very last.

Patients in an apparently moribund state may recover sufficiently to require rehabilitation not only for themselves physically, but also emotionally for their carers, their families and their friends and partners.

Many researchers have studied possible predictive factors for progression from HIV to AIDS and also factors which may predict or determine survival from the first AIDS defining illness to death. It is clear that there are still unknown factors and there appear to be no single markers which give complete certainty. However, a number of markers in combination do give indications as to the progression of the disease.

The patient's morale, sense of control and meaning, his sense of support and his will to live undoubtedly play a part in determining length of survival. Good symptom control, when it significantly improves quality of life, appears to prolong life in some cases, although this is not the prime purpose of symptom control

The use of zidovudine to treat patients with AIDS, and the improved treatments and prophylaxis now available for such conditions as *Pneumocystis carinii* pneumonia, have lengthened median survival times, as was shown in a study conducted at St Mary's Hospital, London (Peters *et al.*, 1991).

A more recent study of CD4 lymphocyte decline has shown that therapy (anti-PCP prophylaxis and/or zidovudine *vs* no therapy) was the single factor most predictive of an increased median survival time, whether total from diagnosis or from the time the patient was found to have a CD4 count of 100. It was concluded that, in the natural history of HIV infection, the CD4 cell decline is predictive of total survival, but that therapy can prolong life and appear to negate the predictive value of CD4 cell decline in survival from CD4 100 to death (Drabbick *et al.*, 1992).

Another multicentre study sought to identify the predictive factors for survival of less than six months or more than two years from an AIDS diagnosis. The findings were that longer survival is associated with higher CD4 cell counts, lymphocyte counts and haemoglobin levels, and lower neopterin (a product of activated macrophages) levels. In this case, age at AIDS diagnosis was not found to affect survival, although other studies have indicated that older patients tend to have shorter survival times (Bogner *et al.*, 1992).

Other markers for disease outcome and progression in HIV infected adults include serum p24, $ß_2$-microglobulin and soluble CD8 antigen concentrations (Siller *et al.*, 1993). Certain opportunistic infections are more likely to develop as the CD4 count declines below 200 (normal above 800/ml). These include cytomegalovirus infection and atypical myobacterial disease. As the CD4 count declines, the number of co-existing diagnoses increases and in end-stage disease, very rapid progression of, for example, KS, or dissemination of infections previously under control by maintenance therapy, may be seen.

In summary, when considering the prognosis of any particular patient, the following points should be borne in mind:

- overall median survival times
- rate of deterioration
- degree of immunosuppression, CD4 count if available
- history of therapy
- constellation of diagnoses and problems
- patient's morale.

Patient-directed care

The advent of AIDS has challenged health care professionals to reexamine their attitudes to those who are in their care. People with AIDS have challenged health care professionals with their intelligent search for a greater understanding of their disease, their need to remain in control, their refusal to be treated as victims or to be 'fobbed off' by ambiguous answers or unclear explanations. The hospice movement and primary carers in the community have, in the past decade or two, led the way in revolutionising the approach to patients from that of 'the doctor knows best' to that of a partnership between the professional and the patient.

What does it mean in practice for the doctor to give control back to the patient and to be involved in patient directed care? It means that clear and honest information is given to patients, enabling them to make their own choices with appropriate guidance from the doctor, but never pressure. It means that the doctor has to accept the patient's choice. It means that the doctor's opinion will often be challenged: the doctor may often find that the patient knows more than the doctor does about his illness. It means that the doctor's opinion may be rejected and recommended medication or advice may not be taken. This can be difficult for the doctor to cope with, particularly when the doctor has been used to being in control and seen as an authority. However, if the doctor sees him or herself as a facilitator, enabler, information and advice giver then there need be no breakdown in the relationship or partnership.

When the patient is confused and demented, who is in control? This issue must be discussed with other team members. The important question here is 'What would the patient have wished had he been able to make a decision?' This question can only be answered through a prior understanding and knowledge of the patient, and the best people to advise are the partner, the family or close friends. They should certainly be involved in decision-making, particularly if the decision involves a major change in management policy.

It is all very well talking about, and seeking to put into practice, patient-directed care when the patient wishes to have control, or is intelligent and able to understand the issues that are involved. It is a different matter to put this into practice when the patient does not wish to make decisions, or is unable to do so, or is manipulative, playing one member of the health care team off against another. In this situation good communication between the members of the interdisciplinary team is of paramount importance. Clear boundaries should be agreed by the team members, who must develop a consistent approach to the patient, keeping each other informed of any developments or changes. It is often useful for two or three members of the caring team, e.g. nurse, doctor and counsellor, to see the patient together when dealing with a difficult issue.

Some patients do not wish to make decisions and may tell the doctor or nurse so. It may be appropriate and necessary for the patient to give the responsibility for decision-making to the professionals for a time, but not usually on a permanent basis. Some may need more time or may simply be unable to make a decision, allowing events to overtake them. This may be a coping mechanism which should be respected; seeking to force a decision from a patient in such a situation may simply result in him withdrawing further. When such tensions arise, it may be appropriate to ask ourselves as professionals 'Who are we treating – the patient or ourselves?'

Active versus palliative care

When is 'active therapy' in fact palliative? In one sense, until there is a definite cure for AIDS, all treatment is palliative. Life-prolonging treatment is, however, clearly available, at least in more affluent countries. Opportunistic infections may be cured or controlled by maintenance therapy until immunosuppression is well advanced. However, in end-stage disease the aim of care must be comfort and quality of life. Good symptom control is essential but in AIDS, it must also be combined with active treatment of, for example, infections which cause debilitating symptoms such as pain or vomiting. Investigations may therefore be necessary to establish a cause when possible; these should only be done in end-stage disease when the management of the problem will be altered by the results or when the patient wishes to have the investigation, if appropriate.

Blood transfusions

The myelosuppressive effects of zidovudine, which is commonly used to slow down the replication of the virus and therefore the progress of the disease, often necessitate the giving of blood transfusions. Severe anaemias may develop, particularly in patients on high doses or who appear to be particularly sensitive. Other myelosuppressive drugs, such as ganciclovir may also contribute. It is clearly appropriate to give blood, when necessary, to someone who is having rehabilitative care, but how appropriate is it to give blood to someone who is terminally ill? In the author's experience the results of blood transfusions in patients who have shown signs of approaching the terminal phase have been disappointing, with very little change in physical energy and any appreciable change lasting, at most, for a couple of weeks. On occasion, there has been a subjective improvement, particularly in the patient's mental state. The decision as to whether or not to give a blood transfusion must be made according to the individual case, and must be made in consultation with the patient who may or may not feel that the trauma of having a blood transfusion is outweighed by the benefits.

Ganciclovir or foscarnet infusions

Ganciclovir or foscarnet infusions are given to prevent the progression of cytomegalovirus (CMV) retinitis to total blindness. Even in the terminal weeks of life progression to blindness may be devastating for the patient, compounding his sense of isolation. It is therefore entirely appropriate, with the patient's cooperation and full understanding, to continue maintenance treatment. Ganciclovir and foscarnet are usually given, through a central line which has been inserted under general or local anaesthesia in hospital, for the initial two to three weeks of treatment (see Chapter 6 for further details). Maintenance treatment is then continued, usually five times a week. If the maintenance therapy is stopped there is an increased risk of reactivation of CMV retinitis with further progression and damage to the eye. When treatment has already been instituted in hospital and maintenance therapy is being given as a matter of course, clearly these treatments should be continued. However, difficult decisions may have to be faced when a patient who may only have weeks to live develops CMV retinitis for the first time.

A patient who on many occasions told the doctor and the nurses that he wished to die and that no active intervention should be made, developed CMV retinitis with what appeared to be only weeks to live. He was already extremely cachetic and weak and could not face further acute treatment, with the transferral to an acute centre, frequent blood tests and daily infusions. His mother agreed with him. However, as his vision deteriorated and he lingered longer than expected, some of the staff found this decision extremely difficult to live with although the patient seemed undistressed. He died three weeks later. His gentle acceptance and quiet withdrawal as death approached made it clear that he was content with his decision, but the difficulty the staff had to face was the uncertainty of his total understanding of the issues involved when he had made the decision, as he was also intermittently confused. The question sometimes has to be asked 'Who would we be treating – the patient, or ourselves and our anxiety?'

Foscarnet is frequently given during the initial treatment phase as a continuous infusion over 24 hours for 3 weeks, followed by maintenance therapy given 5 times a week over 4 to 8 hours. This kind of therapy is very restrictive for the patient and, together with the frequent blood tests that are required to monitor the nephrotoxic effect, may detract considerably from the possible quality of life that is available to the patient. What constitutes quality of life for one patient may be quite different for another and decisions must be made with each individual, and must be regularly reviewed.

Both ganciclovir and foscarnet infusions can be given in the home, provided that either the patient is able to give the infusions himself, or the community nurses are able to take on this task. Patients can be taught to give their own infusions; however this may not be possible for patients developing encephalopathy or other neurological problems, or as their illness progresses and they become weaker.

A patient whose prognosis was extremely uncertain but who had been fairly stable for some months opted for referral from the hospice unit back to his acute centre for insertion of the Hickman line, followed by a return to the hospice for the continuation of the initial treatment and then maintenance therapy. He eventually learnt to give his own infusion and was able to return home for some months.

If home treatment is not possible, a day centre may enable the patient to have the treatment but still live at home.

Total parenteral nutrition (TPN)

Maintenance of total nutrition via a central line is an increasingly popular option for patients suffering from the debilitating effects of persistent severe diarrhoea caused by cryptosporidiosis, together with the nausea and vomiting that often accompanies it. Both the diarrhoea and the vomiting are very resistant to treatment and control may be very difficult to achieve without unacceptable side effects (see also Chapter 6). High standards of aseptic technique are required to prevent infection, regular blood tests once or twice weekly are needed to ensure correct electrolyte and nutritional balance, and close liaison is required between the doctor, the dietitian, the pharmacist who makes up the mixture, and the laboratory services. For the patient with oesophageal KS or intractable vomiting and diarrhoea, but whose prognosis is otherwise reasonably good, this may be a viable option. It then becomes a life-line, and the question arises as to when this life-line should be cut. This may be an enormously difficult question for both the patient and his family to cope with and it may, indeed, never be faced, either by them or by the doctors and nurses involved. Since it is the nurses who generally set up the TPN and who are more intimately involved with the patient they may well be the first to ask the question; and they may be the best people to begin the discussion with the patient or the family.

Total parental nutrition can, of course, be given at home or in the community, provided there is someone trained and able to maintain the high aseptic standards that are required in giving the daily infusion. The general practitioner or home care team and dietitian will have to liaise closely with laboratory services and pharmacists to ensure successful continuation of this therapy, which requires a high level of commitment by all.

Investigations

Some investigations involve quite traumatic procedures. In the case of the patient who is having rehabilitative or convalescent care and is not yet obviously terminally ill, it is clear that any sudden deterioration or change should be investigated, and decisions have to be made about where these investigations should take place. However, when somebody has entered the terminal phase of the illness, the question should be asked, 'Who will benefit from this investigation? What change in management will be indicated by the result of the investigation?' In other words, if the result of any investigation is likely to substantially alter the management, then it is appropriate for the investigation to be done. However, if the investigation is merely for academic satisfaction then it may be quite inappropriate to subject either the patient or his family to the trauma involved in taking blood tests, performing lumbar punctures etc. Of course it is important to add to the total knowledge that we have about AIDS, but this need has to be balanced against the rights and needs of the patient.

Protection for the doctor and other health care professionals

All body fluids should be treated with circumspection, whether they are known or not to come from someone who is HIV positive. Gloves should be worn by anyone coming into contact with body fluids or at risk of doing so, and a plastic apron worn to protect clothes. Gloves should also be worn by anyone taking blood, and of course whenever intravenous injections or infusions are set up. These same standards should ideally be applied wherever care is being given, not only to people known to have AIDS but to all categories of patients, and all blood should be treated as potentially infected, either with hepatitis B or HIV. Further information is given in Chapter 4 under 'Infection control'.

Radiotherapy and chemotherapy

In the terminal phases of advanced AIDS, radiotherapy may be appropriate to provide palliation for a severely swollen limb as a result of KS, and chemotherapy may reduce oesophageal obstruction caused by KS and may also reduce pain associated with swallowing. However, again side effects may outweigh the benefits and decisions may have to be made regarding the continuation of or the stopping of therapy. These decisions cannot be arrived at without discussion of all the available options and possible outcomes.

A patient admitted for terminal care with KS involving most of the lower lobe of the right lung regained his determination and will to live to such an extent that he was prepared to undergo radiotherapy to his lung and to several skin lesions to a total of 13 treatments. Each of these involved an ambulance trip across London to the radiotherapy centre in the referring hospital. The patient was warned that the prognosis for someone with KS lung was usually a matter of weeks and at best with radiotherapy a few months, at most six or seven. Two and a half months after admission he was discharged to sheltered accommodation where he lived with his partner with considerable quality of life for a further six months.

For this patient the benefits of treatment far outweighed the disadvantages, but for others it does not.

A patient with the same problem as mentioned above opted to have no active intervention, but accepted symptom control measures which made him very comfortable and enabled him to live the final three or four weeks of his life with great zest and enjoyment, in spite of the increasing dyspnoea and general weakness. He preferred to conserve his energies for settling his affairs, being reconciled with his family, and meeting Her Royal Highness, The Princess of Wales when she visited the hospice unit.

When death approaches

In most cases it is clear to all involved with a patient that he is deteriorating. However, as has already been said, it is extremely risky to prognosticate as patients often have a very strong will and determination to live. In the author's experience some patients have clung on to their regular daily dosages of zidovudine until the day they died; some, as illustrated by the case histories given here, have confounded all prognostications, recovered against all odds and have been able to go home, albeit for a short while. However, there comes a time when it is evident that the patient is entering the terminal phase and probably has only a few days to live – when the patient has become increasingly weak and immobile, is less interested in food and drink, spends much of the day sleeping or drowsy, and may have developed signs of an early broncho-pneumonia. The question then arises, 'Who do you tell and how much?' The patient is usually aware and may or may not wish to speak about his situation. The partner and family or close friends are anxious to know 'How long?' and 'What will happen?' It should never be acceptable to say there is nothing more that can be done, to say that those responsible for providing care have given up. *There is always something more that can be done to ensure the patient's comfort and ease from distress.*

The family need to be aware that the patient may linger for several days longer than expected. During this time the family may wish to see the doctor frequently and will certainly require a great deal of support and comfort from the nursing and other staff. The family require reassurance that the patient will not suffer; with good symptom control this assurance can be given with confidence.

How much do you tell? The answer to this question depends to some extent on your relationship with the family and friends and with the patient. It is important that all members of the team know what is being said and discussed and that those who are close to the patient are not given conflicting information. It is also sometimes important to spare them from unnecessarily distressing details.

A patient developed CMV retinitis within days of death. It was obvious to the hospice staff that the patient was becoming blind, but they felt that it was an unnecessarily distressing detail with which to burden the mother, especially as the patient seemed not to be distressed.

The doctor's role in terminal care

Within the multiprofessional team the doctor must work in close cooperation with the nursing team, listening to them as well as to the patient and those who are close to him. As has already been suggested, the nurses provide the most intimate care and spend the longest time with the patient, so are in an ideal position to observe and understand the needs of the patient. The doctor is one member of the full multiprofessional team and must also liaise closely with chaplains, physiotherapists, occupational therapists and counsellors, as well as social workers or others involved. He or she must also maintain contact with and liaise with consultants and other doctors who have been involved in the patient's care so that appropriate and coordinated care is given on a continuing basis. During the final few days it is the doctor's duty to monitor closely the results of symptom control measures, together with the nurses involved and then to certify death when this occurs.

After death the family continues to require support, but the doctor's role here is clearly to deal with such practical matters such as the death certificate, cremation form and autopsies where appropriate as quickly and as efficiently as possible. It is important to have thought through the whole issue of what goes on the death certificate before the actual time comes when the certificate has to be written. The word 'AIDS' on a death certificate can cause a tremendous amount of trauma to the family, as death certificates are not private property and are available for inspection by a number of bodies. It is acceptable to write only the immediate and obvious cause of death, such as broncho-pneumonia or viral encephalitis with associated causes of death such as CMV infection, mycobacterial disease etc., on the death certificate. In the UK there is a box on the back of the form which may be ticked, offering further information. A confidential letter should also be sent to the doctor or person whose responsibility it is to collect statistical information about the causes of death in the country, giving the full details of the diagnosis. Cremation forms in Britain should have the same wording as on the death certificate.

The educational needs of the doctor

Doctors who are involved in terminal and continuing care for people with AIDS are privileged to share in the darkness (see Dr Sheila Cassidy's (1988) book, *Sharing the Darkness*), but also in some of the trials, and even joys, that the patient and those close to him will be going through. It is, inevitably, a time of deep sadness and trauma for all involved. All those involved in the patient's care will be looking to the doctor for guidance and for information about the cause of the disease, about its management, about the prognosis, and for the symptom control. It is vitally important that the doctor is fully aware of the progress of the disease. It is also very important that doctors keep up to date with current knowledge, maintain close contacts with colleagues and other sources of information about the current state of research into new drugs, vaccines and other therapies. If doctors do not have the knowledge themselves, they should at least know where to turn for information and advice.

Support for doctors

Doctors do not only need to keep up to date clinically. Anyone involved in the care of people with life-threatening illnesses will be aware that he or she will frequently face deep searching questions, and difficult dilemmas. Doctors may find that their beliefs or world views are seriously challenged, and experience the emotional draining that comes with multiple bereavement. It is therefore important that doctors recognise their own needs in terms of support. This support may be available through the multiprofessional team, through colleagues, family or other support networks such as church or friends. Individuals will have their own support network. If doctors are to continue to provide effective support to the patients and their families during this special, but very traumatic, time and afterwards, they must ensure that they have support for themselves.

References

Bogner, J.R., Sadri, I., Schreiber, M.A. *et al.* (1992) Uncommon courses of AIDS: differences between patients with very short and very long survival. AIDS Forschung **7** (7): 347–50.

Drabbick, J.J., Williams, W.J., Tang, D.B. *et al.* (1992). CD4 lymphocyte decline and survival in human immuno-deficiency virus infection. *AIDS Research*, **8(12)**, 2039–47.

Peters, R.S., Beck, E.J., Coleman, D.G. *et al.* (1991). Changing disease patterns in patients with AIDS in a referral centre in The UK: the changing face of AIDS. Brit. Med. Journal **302**, 203–7.

Siller, L., Martin, N.L., Kostuchenko, P. *et al.* (1993). Serum levels of soluble CD8, neopterin, β_2-microglobulin and p24 antigen as indicators of disease progression in children with AIDS on zidovudine therapy. *AIDS*, **7** 369–73.

6

Symptom control and common medical problems

' . . . meticulous attention to detail can lead to appropriate and
effective treatment to the end of a patient's life. This transforms his
experience, and the memories of his family.'

Dame Cicely Saunders in Twycross and Lack (1990)

The above quotation from Dame Cicely Saunders' foreword to the well
known book *Therapeutics in Terminal Cancer* is equally true for the care of
patients with advanced AIDS. A conversation overheard in the street,
where one woman was saying to another 'The doctor said there was
nothing more they could do for him . . . ' is still sadly the experience of
many people. In terms of a cure, it is of course true that there comes a
time when nothing more can be done to achieve a cure, or to prolong life
with quality. However, it is never true that nothing more can be done to
make a patient more comfortable.

This chapter is set in the context of a book which seeks throughout to
deal with the needs of the whole person. Good medical management
and symptom control is only one aspect of the whole. However, it is an
aspect of care which may profoundly affect the experience of the
patient, and the memories with which the partners, families or friends
have to live for many years to follow. Their memories may also
profoundly affect their own attitudes to facing issues of death and
dying.

A patient with severe peripheral neuropathy, which was
proving difficult to control, was found, on probing more
deeply, to have vivid memories of his father's problems with
severe diabetic neuropathy and eventual bilateral above knee
amputations prior to his death. These memories were very

frightening and undoubtedly affected his own reaction to the peripheral neuropathy that he was experiencing.

Of necessity, this chapter must be brief in giving only an overview of the way in which advanced AIDS presents in the terminal care situation. It gives a description of the common symptoms encountered, guide-lines for dealing with them, and some comments about common medical problems which may present management difficulties. It is based on the experience gained since February 1988 when Mildmay opened its hospice unit for people with AIDS. It was the first such unit in Europe and therefore had no model to follow. The principles of palliative care in cancer gave us our basic guidelines but much of our learning as a team was experiential. We learned from and with each other, but most of all we learnt from and with our patients.

Good symptom control in advanced AIDS depends on the following:

Attention to detail It is important to invest time to examine the patient in detail and to listen carefully to his description of his problems and symptoms. Careful assessment of the degree to which a symptom is felt should also be made; this is particularly relevant in dealing with a symptom such as pain where good control will depend on meticulous monitoring of the response to therapy. It is important to bear in mind that significant changes can take place very rapidly in a patient with AIDS and that the doctor's perception of a problem may differ considerably from that of the patient himself.

Good *liaison* and *communication* between nurses and doctors. Nurses are the people who spend most time with the patient, and are involved in many intimate procedures which mean that they are in an excellent position to observe and monitor symptoms and the result of medication. Many nurses are skilled listeners and observers, and often the patients will discuss details with the nurses that they would not talk about with the doctor.

A good *knowledge* and *understanding* of:

● AIDS and its presentation in the advanced stages of the disease
● the drugs commonly used in the treatment of AIDS and related problems
● the therapeutic principles of palliative medicine, e.g. pain control.

Many good books have been written about the basic principles of terminal care in cancer and other life threatening illnesses to which reference should also be made. This chapter will deal with the differences encountered in caring for someone with AIDS, although there are, of course, some overlapping areas of care which will also be dealt with briefly where appropriate. (See the Introduction for a list of differences.)

The patient

Patients with AIDS cannot and should not be categorised and grouped. Nor is it possible to describe any one particular type of patient. Chapter 2 described, in the authors' experience, some of the main differences encountered in patients with AIDS, compared with those having cancer. However, it must be remembered that this experience is limited by location in the West and in a large cosmopolitan capital city. It is, nevertheless, true to say that people with AIDS will, in the main, be young people, many of them in what should be the prime of their lives. The majority of people with AIDS, in the West, apart from children or people with haemophilia, will be in the age range of 20–49 years.

Multiple diagnoses and inevitable polypharmacy

All patients with AIDS will have a number of co-existing diagnoses, many of which will be opportunistic infections for which the patient will be receiving active treatment, maintenance therapy for control of persisting problems, or prophylaxis to prevent recurrence of opportunistic infections.

Many patients will also require drugs related specifically to symptom control. Some symptoms, for example nausea and vomiting, might be directly related to the drugs the patient is taking. Other symptoms such as pain or parathesiae, dysphagia, or diarrhoea might be due to the effects of the HIV virus itself, or of opportunistic infections. Although the number of drugs that a patient may be taking might be rationalised, and in some cases reduced, the doctor is often forced into practising polypharmacy in trying to control or prevent the recurrence of distressing or painful conditions such as herpes simplex or a life-threatening condition such as cerebral toxoplasmosis or *Pneumocystis carinii* pneumonia (PCP). The time will inevitably come when it is appropriate to stop prophylactic treatment; this is obvious when the patient has become unconscious or is no longer able to take oral medications, but not so obvious when the patient is still conscious and anxious about the possible onset, for example, of PCP or dementia. Such decisions have to be made in discussions with the patient, with where possible explanation of the likely outcomes. Some patients for example, find acyclovir difficult to swallow, and although there are few side effects, patients will often opt to stop this drug. Septrin is another tablet that many dislike taking. Most of the antituberculous drugs are also difficult to take and cause nausea and vomiting; many patients improve subjectively on stopping these medications. Robert's story at the beginning of Chapter 5 illustrates a number of these points.

Common conditions and infections found in advanced HIV disease

This section does not attempt or pretend to be an exhaustive introduction to clinical aspects of AIDS. It is intended to provide the general practitioner, hospice doctor, or other health care professional involved with a terminally ill AIDS patient, with a brief introduction to the conditions and infections most likely to be encountered. Where appropriate the prognostic significance of certain conditions is indicated and information on available treatment options given. Readers who wish to know more about AIDS and its many complex manifestations, its immunology and epidemiology should refer to the many good text books and journals that are available (see 'Further reading').

Introduction

The progression of HIV infection to AIDS goes through a number of stages which will be briefly described.

Acute seroconversion illness

Two to six weeks after initial infection some people develop a short, 'flu-like' illness with fever, arthralgia and, in some instances, a maculopapular rash. Some also develop lymphadenopathy which resolves within weeks. There is some evidence that the severity of the fever and rash, in particular, is a prognostic marker for more rapid progression to AIDS. It is at this stage that individuals become antibody positive, i.e. they start producing antibodies to HIV.

Antibody positive: asymptomatic

Individuals may remain asymptomatic but antibody positive on testing for a variable number of years. These individuals are infected and carry the virus; they are therefore infectious to others through the normal routes of transmission.

Antibody positive: symptomatic

As the infection progresses, the CD4 lymphocyte count declines and eventually patients begin to develop signs of ill health. These may include non-specific problems such as fatigue, anorexia, weight loss, persistent lymphadenopathy and diarrhoea. Bacterial and fungal skin infections, seborrhoeic dermatitis, herpes simplex and zoster infections and oral candidiasis may occur from time to time. Some patients continue to deteriorate and become chronically debilitated even though they have not yet developed any AIDS-defining conditions. During this time the CD4 count continues to decline and antigen levels rise, although there is not usually a smooth progression. (See also Chapter 5, 'Prognosis').

AIDS

AIDS is diagnosed when one or more conditions develop which are considered by the Centers for Disease Control to be 'AIDS defining'. As more becomes known about HIV/AIDS, the list is updated from time to time and may differ in minor details in America, Europe and other parts of the world. These conditions include certain opportunistic infections, AIDS-related cancers and HIV encephalopathy (or dementia). (See Table 10.)

Common opportunistic infections

The primary cause of morbidity and mortality in patients with AIDS is opportunistic infections. The following points should be borne in mind when caring for an AIDS patient:

- Because of immunosuppression the presentation of an opportunistic infection may be unusual.
- For the same reason infections may present as, or become, disseminated.
- Complete cure is often not possible, although good response to treatment of an acute episode may be obtained. Long-term suppressive or maintenance therapy is often required.
- A number of different infections may co-exist or occur at the same time.
- Most opportunistic infections, such as cytomegalovirus infections, tuberculosis, toxoplasmosis and possibly *Pneumocystis carinii* pneumonia, are the result of re-activation of latent, previously acquired infections.
- Primary prophylaxis against infections such as *Pneumocystis carinii* may improve survival.
- Opportunistic infections commonly occur in patients whose CD4 count is below 200–300/ml.

Pneumocystis carinii *pneumonia* (PCP)

This is the most common AIDS-defining illness in Western countries with 60 per cent of patients presenting with PCP. It occurs once or more in 80 per cent of patients with AIDS (Polis and Masur, 1989) although this pattern may change as some patients are offered primary prophylaxis against PCP. *Pneumocystis carinii* is thought to be a fungus which is part of the normal flora of most adults. PCP is uncommon in Africa (Abonya *et al.*, 1992) although it is found in the environment. The *presentation* may be acute with severe respiratory distress, fever and an extremely ill patient. In the early part of the 1980s, such patients would often be managed on a ventilator, but this is now unusual. Most patients (90 per cent) will now survive this first episode of PCP. Improved survival is thought to be partly due to the use of steroids in the acute episode.

Some patients present with a 3–4 week history of a dry cough and increasing dyspnoea. Chest X-rays may be inconclusive or show diffuse alveolar and interstitial infiltration. Diagnosis is made by induced sputum, bronchoalveolar lavage or biopsy and microscopic demonstration of the organisms. Patients who have been on prophylaxis, or whose immunosuppression is well-advanced, may present few obvious signs or symptoms. In terminally ill patients with end-stage disease it would be inappropriate to perform invasive investigations and treatment should be aimed at achieving comfort.

Treatment is usually with trimethoprim-sulphamethoxazole (cotrimoxazole) 6–8 hourly, in high doses, either intravenously or orally for three weeks, or with IV pentamidine (see Table 13 for dosages and side effects). Co-trimoxazole frequently causes a severe rash and anaemia, but it has been found to be more effective than pentamidine in severe infections (Polis and Masur, 1989; Martin *et al.*, 1992). Pentamidine is nephrotoxic and may cause hypoglycaemia and hypotension. In less severe infections pentamidine may be given by nebuliser or co-trimoxazole orally; PCP may then be managed on an outpatient basis. Co-trimoxazole is the drug of choice for prophylaxis; pentamidine by nebuliser every 2–4 weeks is also effective, although some people find it unpleasant. Bronchospasm may be a problem; salbutamol is usually given prior to pentamidine administration.

Other treatments which may be used for PCP treatment or prophylaxis include dapsone, pyrimethamine with sulphadoxine (Fansidar) or clindamycin with primaquine. Dapsone has recently been shown to be as effective as pentamidine for prophylaxis, but causes fewer side effects and is less expensive and easier to administer (Slavin *et al.*, 1992 – see also Table 13 for drug dosages, side effects and interactions).

Cytomegalovirus (CMV)

CMV is a member of the herpes group of viruses and is widely spread through the general population with particularly high prevalence rates in densely populated areas. Congenital CMV infections may cause serious neurological problems but acquired infection in adults only rarely cause serious illness. However in AIDS, where HIV causes a deficiency in cell-mediated immunity, CMV infections are associated with disseminated disease affecting many organs. CMV is commonly associated with PCP and may also cause encephalitis, colitis or oesophagitis. However the most serious effect is on the retina where it causes *retinitis* which, if left untreated, may progress rapidly to total blindness. Patients admitted for long term terminal care should be examined every few weeks for signs of CMV retinitis as it may initially be asymptomatic. The patient may complain simply of blurring of vision or have noticed recent problems with peripheral vision. Examination of the fundi may reveal signs of acute retinitis including haemorrhages (said to resemble a cheese and tomato pizza), but the patient should, in any case of doubt be referred for immediate ophthalmological opinion. It is often unilateral and even if only partial vision is possible in one eye, the other eye may be spared by treatment and maintenance therapy (ganciclovir or foscarnet by infusion via a central or Hickman line). CMV *oesophagitis, colitis* and *hepatitis* are less common (see Table 13.) CMV oesophagitis causes severe burning retro-sternal pain with dysphagia, and CMV colitis causes a watery diarrhoea which may be profuse, and occasionally causes fresh bleeding. It may be accompanied by abdominal pain and distension; occasionally perforation of the bowel may occur. There may be fever and, inevitably, weight loss. Foscarnet or ganciclovir infusions may be successful in reducing the volume of diarrhoea and in improving the general condition of the patient. Sadly, some CMV infections become resistant to these anti-viral agents, and will re-activate in spite of continuing maintenance therapy. Alternating treatment courses may reduce this likelihood.

In a comparative study of clinical and autopsy diagnosis in Italy, it was found that CMV visceral infection accounted for the majority of diseases not recognised in life. Single organs infected but not diagnosed in life included the adrenal gland, the lung, the brain and the gastro-intestinal tract, but disseminated infections involving several organs were also found, though more likely to have been diagnosed in life (Monforte *et al.*, 1992) (see Table 13 for dosage regimes).

Toxoplasmosis

This is caused by the protozoan *Toxoplasma gondii* which infects humans after ingestion of cysts in infected meat or cat faeces. Released from the cysts in the gastrointestinal tract, the active tachyzoites enter the blood stream via the gastric mucosa and spread to all tissues in the body, but particularly to the brain, although disseminated infection may affect the heart, liver, lungs and spleen where abscesses may form. Focal neurological problems are the commonest signs of development. The diagnosis is made by CT or MRI scan and active treatment instituted, although brain biopsy is required for definitive diagnosis. Most patients remain on prophylaxis following initial treatment.

Most centres will now give a trial of *treatment* without proceeding to brain biopsy. Initial treatment is pyrimethamine (75 mg loading dose, then 25 mg od) with sulphadiazine (1 g 6-hourly) and folinic acid (15 mg daily) for 3–6 weeks, with a CT or MRI scan at three weeks to monitor response. A prompt response is usual, with clinical improvement in 90 per cent of patients who have toxoplasmosis. *Maintenance* therapy is then required with pyrimethamine 25 mg od, sulphadiazine 500–1000 mg od or bd, with folinic acid. Patients who develop side effects may be treated with clindamycin and pyrimethamine or Atovaquone which has recently been found to be effective and is well tolerated (Kovacs *et al.*, 1992). Pyrimethamine alone, at 50 mg daily, has also been shown to be effective as maintenance therapy.

In patients with *end-stage disease*, toxoplasmosis that has been suppressed may recur causing focal neurological problems with headache, nausea and confusion. Symptoms may improve for some time if the patient is treated with dexamethasone, but it must of course be borne in mind that the progression of the toxoplasmosis or other opportunistic infections may then be masked. Toxoplasmosis may also occur in other forms, although this not so common – retinochoroiditis, pneumonitis and orchitis have been reported.

Mycobacterial disease

Mycobacterial disease in general is more common in patients with AIDS than in other patients. *Mycobacterium tuberculosis* causes typical pulmonary disease which may or may not be resistant to treatment, depending on geographical area and resistance patterns. Atypical mycobacteria are frequently resistant to most conventional drug regimes. MAI is a complex of two strains, *Mycobacterium avium* and *Mycobacterium intracellulare* and has been found in approximately 50 per cent of AIDS patients at post mortem. Other atypical mycobacteria are found in AIDS, for example *M. xenopi* and *M. kanasaii*. MAI is the most common form found in the UK and usually causes disseminated disease affecting the gut, bone marrow, liver, lung, spleen, adrenal glands, brain, lymph nodes and kidney. *Diagnosis* is made by finding acid-fast bacilli and culturing appropriate samples. *Treatment* is with anti-tuberculous medication such as a combination of, for example, Rifambutin, ethambutol, pyrazinamide, and isoniazid. These commonly cause side effects such as nausea and vomiting and, as the patient's general condition deteriorates, some patients may opt to stop treatment. This may be appropriate in patients when the emphasis of care is on quality of life. However, many patients experience severe symptoms of fever and night sweats when treatment is stopped. There is evidence of increasing incidence of multidrug resistance and there is concern about the possibilities of nosocomial infections in clinics and inpatient facilities where patients with open pulmonary tuberculosis may congegate (Beck-Sague *et al.*, 1992).

Patients with disseminated MAI who are nearing the terminal phase frequently experience increasing fatigue, anorexia, weight loss with diarrhoea and may become severely anaemic. Blood transfusion may only give symptomatic relief for 2–3 weeks, if at all. Anaemia may recur within two weeks and it may then be inappropriate to continue to give transfusions. Supportive care, with an emphasis on quality and symptom control, becomes more important.

On laparotomy, prior to admission, a patient was found to have disseminated abdominal tuberculosis and opted to stop all anti-tuberculous medication. Soon after admission for terminal care he developed symptoms and signs of an acute abdomen. He chose to remain at the hospice, and was started on 8 mg of dexamethasone daily which was gradually reduced over a period of weeks to 1 mg daily. He recovered rapidly from his acute abdomen and his general condition improved so that over a period of time he was able to go home every weekend and after several months went home to stay with his parents where he lived until he died almost a year after his initial admission. The patient continued to refuse anti-tuberculous medication, and was maintained throughout on either 0.5 or 1 mg of dexamethasone. Attempts at stopping this always resulted in a recurrence of symptoms and a deterioration in his general well-being. Six months prior to his death he also developed CMV retinitis, and did opt to have a Hickman line inserted and intravenous ganciclovir therapy. He retained the vision of one eye but lost most effective vision in the other. The patient eventually succumbed to disseminated mycobacterial disease.

Cryptosporidial and other diarrhoeas

Cryptosporidium muris is a parasite which causes damage to the gastro-intestinal mucosa, with fusion of villi and production of a profuse watery diarrhoea, sometimes amounting to 8–10 litres per day. It is usually accompanied by abdominal pain, loud borborygmi and flatulence, severe general malaise and loss of weight, with malabsorption. There may be fever, and in some patients nausea and vomiting are a prominent feature. Even when the cryptosporidiosis has been successfully treated, which is frequently not possible, the patient may be left with permanent mucosal damage leading to diarrhoea and continued malabsorption. A very large number of drugs have been tried in an attempt to treat this infection, but none with any significant degree of success although occasional individuals have responded to *treatment*. In the *terminal care situation* diarrhoea should be controlled as far as possible with oral rehydration fluid, antidiarrhoeal and antiemetic drugs, as well as, where possible, treatment of the cause. In cryptosporidiosis it is usually effective to start with loperamide 4–8 mg qds (up to maximum of 32 mg in 24 hours – above the usual recommended dose, but safe with no CNS effects). The addition of isphaghula in the form of Fybogel twice or three times daily will thicken the stool and an antispasmodic such as Buscopan (hyoscine butyl bromide) may also help. Constipation is not likely to occur, even with regular medication, and for some patients it is necessary to use opiates. Once it has been decided to use opiate medication, the appropriate dosage should be titrated in the normal way using 4-hourly morphine or diamorphine initially orally, until some success in controlling the diarrhoea has been achieved, then changing to 12-hourly dosages of sustained release morphine sulphate tablets for convenience. In a patient who has intractable vomiting, diamorphine in a syringe driver may be very effective in combination with an antiemetic such as metoclopramide, haloperidol or, in severe cases, methotrimeprazine. It is not always possible to prevent the diarrhoea completely; however it has been possible to reduce the frequency of diarrhoea from perhaps 10, 12 or more times to 3 or 4 times in 24 hours, sometimes down to 1 or 2. Stool volumes may continue to be large even at this frequency.

It is becoming more common to give *parenteral nutrition* through a Hickman central line to patients with the severe weight loss and wasting that is associated with this kind of diarrhoea. TPN is also given to patients with oesophageal obstruction as a result of KS or lymphoma. Weekly or twice weekly blood tests are necessary to ensure electrolyte and nutritional balance, and close liaison is required between doctors, the dietitian, the pharmacist and the laboratory services. Meticulous aseptic techniques must be maintained by those who are involved in

Table 2. Control of nausea, vomiting and diarrhoea in cryptosporidiosis

Symptom	Recommended therapy
Nausea/vomiting	Metoclopramide* po/IM 10–20 mg tds Cyclizine* po/IM/PR 25–50 mg tds Haloperidol* po/s–c 0.5–5 mg bd possibly Nabilone po 1–2 mg bd
Intractable vomiting	*via syringe driver if necessary; or methotrimeprazine starting with 25–50 mg over 12 hours Sometimes two or more required in combination
Diarrhoea	Loperamide 4–8 mg qds (max. 32 mg in 24 hours) Fybogel 1–3 sachets daily
Intractable diarrhoea	Morphine/diamorphine po or s–c by syringe driver (titrate dose in usual way) (see also text)

Note: Higher dosages may be necessary.
Persistent nausea or diarrhoea should not be treated in a prn basis.

setting up the daily TPN (usually the nurse but patients may also learn to do this themselves to maintain independence – see also Chapter 5).

Table 2 suggests the recommended therapy for the control of nausea, vomiting and diarrhoea in cryptosporidiosis. Recent reports suggest that paromomycin may be useful in the treatment of intestinal cryptosporidiosis. Patients treated with 500 mg 6-hourly po usually respond with a decrease in diarrhoea, stabilisation of weight and, in some, eradication of cryptosporidia from the stool, although relapses do occur. Paromomycin, which is not absorbed systemically, is well tolerated (Fitchenbaum et al., 1993).

Other pathogens which cause diarrhoea include Entamoeba histolytica, Giardia lamblia, shigella, salmonella, campylobacter, Isospora belli, microsporidia, CMV and MAI. Where possible, appropriate treatment of the organism should be given, with symptom control measures as necessary (see later under 'Common symptoms and their control', and also Table 2).

Candida albicans

Candida albicans is the most common cause of mouth problems in HIV disease. It manifests itself through inflammation and soreness with the typical white plaques of oral thrush which, when severe, may coat the tongue, the hard and soft palate, the mucosal lining and gums and may also spread into the pharynx. Candida albicans may affect the whole of the gastro-intestinal tract, and commonly also affects the oesophagus.

Table 3. Common oral conditions, other than *Candida albicans*

Condition	Treatment/comment
Hairy leucoplakia (white adherent patches on sides of tongue associated with Epstein–Barr virus)	Seldom causes problems, therefore treatment is not usually necessary
Gingivitis and dental abscesses	Dental advice and good oral hygiene
Herpes simplex Stomatitis Oesophageal ulceration	Acyclovir 200–400 mg × 5 per day Acyclovir IV
CMV infection; oral or oesophageal ulceration	May respond to IV ganciclovir or foscarnet
Aphthous ulceration	Hydrocortisone 2.5 mg lozenges Betamethasone 0.1 mg pellets (both applied directly to the ulcer) if very painful and extensive– Benzydamine (Difflam) mouthwash; Thalidomide 50–100 mg daily

The symptoms vary from dryness or soreness of the mouth to severe retro-sternal discomfort and dysphagia. Until recently ketoconazole has been the drug of choice for *treatment* and *prophylaxis*. The drugs itraconazole and fluconazole, both of which are less hepatotoxic and cause fewer side effects, have now become more popular. Fluconazole may be given as a single oral daily dose; 150 mg daily for 5–7 days is usually sufficient to control an exacerbation. Many patients are prescribed fluconazole 50–100 mg daily or 2–3 times weekly to maintain control. It has been shown to be more effective than ketoconazole (Laine *et al.*, 1992). However, in patients with far advanced disease, the infection may become resistant to treatment. Oesophageal candidiasis causes dysphagia and retrosternal discomfort, with nausea and retching or vomiting and consequent weight loss. It may require treatment with 200 mg fluconazole bd or with itraconazole. Clotrimazole (vaginal) tablets, 500 mg, if sucked once or twice daily will quickly clear resistant oral thrush; they do not taste very good, but the results are usually worthwhile, (see also p. 127ff.).

When a patient is unable to take tablets, and in the terminal situation, it is usually possible to continue treatment with nystatin oral suspension, given every 2–4 hours. In immunocompromised debilitated patients or children it may also be made up and frozen as iceballs or ice lollies to be sucked. In immunocompromised patients higher doses may be required than those recommended by the manufacturers (Meunier-Carpentier, 1984). Some people dislike the taste and prefer to suck pastilles of nystatin or amphotericin lozenges. However, these do tend

Table 4. Herpes infections

Condition	Treatment
Herpes simplex*	
Stomatitis	Acyclovir 200–400 mg × 5 per day
Oesophageal ulcer	IV acyclovir
Anorectal herpes simplex (may cause severe tenesmus)	Acyclovir 200–400 mg × 5 per day × 5 days
	Acyclovir cream × 5 per day
Herpes simplex on penis or scrotum	Acyclovir 200–400 mg × 5 per day × 5 days
	Acyclovir cream × 5 per day
Herpes zoster*	
Chickenpox or shingles in one or more dermatomes	Acyclovir 800 mg × 5 per day × 7 days
Post herpetic neuralgia	Carbamazepine, also clonazepam in some cases
Ophthalmic or neurological complications	IV acyclovir and specialist supervision

Note: * Risk of meningitis or encephalitis if left untreated or not taking prophylaxis following first infection.

to make the mouth feel dry and furred and, in someone who is becoming dehydrated as a result of reduced oral intake, this can be a problem. Good oral hygiene with regular chlorhexidine mouthwashes or gel may be as important as medication. Table 3 indicates other common oral conditions with which the AIDS patient may present.

Herpes infections

Herpes simplex infections are very common and cause oral or oesophageal ulceration, or ano-rectal and genital problems with ulceration and pain (see Table 4). Oral and oesophageal ulceration has been dealt with above; ano-rectal and genital herpes simplex infections are particularly common in homosexual patients. In ano-rectal herpes infection, defaecation is usually very painful with severe tenesmus. *Treatments* of 400 mg of acyclovir 5 times daily for 5 days may be very effective in dealing both with the infection and the pain. After cleaning with normal saline, acyclovir cream applied to the perianal area or to ulcers on the penis or scrotum, will ease the symptoms and promote healing (see also p. 128–9).

Herpes zoster causing chickenpox or shingles, is said to occur in up to 50 per cent of patients with HIV disease. Shingles is a common sign of immunosuppression and in HIV disease may present in more than one dermatome, or may recur. Post-herpetic neuralgia may persist and require treatment with, for example, carbamazepine. There is a risk of herpes zoster meningitis and patients are usually given acyclovir prophylactically.

Cryptococcal disease

Cryptococcal disease is caused by the yeast *Cryptococcus neoformans* and is the second most common opportunistic neurological infection, after toxoplasmosis, in the Western setting. Meningitis is its most common presentation, but the cryptococcus may also involve heart, lungs, gastrointestinal tract, bone marrow, blood, joints, eyes, skin and lymphatic system.

The *onset* of meningitis may be insidious with low-grade fever and persistent headaches, but it may also have a more acute presentation with obvious signs of meningitis. Amphotericin B and 5-flucytosine were the standard *treatment*, but more recently fluconazole, either intravenously or orally, has been found to be effective. Patients will require continuing prophylaxis with fluconazole 200–400 mg daily or bd. Relapses are not unusual.

In the *terminal care* setting, where the patient may have opted for no further active intervention, the aim of care will be comfort and symptom control as required. Headache and vomiting may be problematic. Headaches may be responsive to codeine phosphate 60 mg 6-hourly (usually more effective than morphine, although this may help more with anxiety). In some instances, where vomiting is a problem, better symptom control will be achieved using a syringe driver with diamorphine and methotrimeprazine (see 'Symptom control', p. 87). Diazepam given rectally will reduce neck stiffness, retraction and muscle tension (10 mg 6-hourly or more frequently may be necessary). Dexamethasone may be effective in reducing symptoms but the disease will of course progress.

Progressive multifocal leucoencephalopathy (PML)

PML is a sub-acute demyelinating disease of the central nervous system and is caused by the papovaviruses JC and SV-40. It has been described in a number of conditions in which cell-mediated immunity is impaired. PML causes multiple lesions in the white matter of the cerebrum producing focal neurological signs. Lesions may also occur in the brain stem and cerebellum. It is rapidly progressive and no treatment has been found to be effective. *Signs* and *symptoms* of the disease may be focal neurological problems, ataxia, mental deterioration and even

Table 5. Neurological conditions in HIV disease (from Youle *et al.*, 1988, *AIDS: Therapeutics in HIV Disease.* Churchill Livingstone)

Human immunodeficiency virus	
Seroconversion illness	Encephalitis
	Meningitis .
	Myelitis
	Nerve palsies
Chronic manifestations	Encephalopathy
	Recurrent meningitis
	Vacuolar myelopathy
	Peripheral neuropathy
	Autonomic neuropathy
Other infections	
Toxoplasma gondii	Cerebral abscesses
Cytomegalovirus	Retinitis, encephalitis
Cryptococcus neoformans	Meningitis
Papovavirus	Progressive multifocal
	leucoencephalopathy (PML)
Mycobacterium tuberculosis	Meningitis, cerebral abscesses
Herpes zoster	Meningitis, Ramsey–Hunt syndrome
Candida albicans	Cerebral abscesses
Nocardia asteroides	Cerebral abscesses
Tumours	
Primary CNS lymphoma	Space-occupying lesion

cortical blindness and paralysis. The *prognosis* is often poor, with death occurring usually within weeks or months after diagnosis (by CT scan and/or brain biopsy). HIV infection may also cause leucoencephalopathy, often producing a similar picture.

Neurological problems related to HIV

HIV itself is known to be neurotropic, but patients with AIDS are also subject to a number of other neurological problems, mostly associated with infections, or tumours. Post-mortem findings indicate that a high proportion of patients develop minor or major neurological disease. Lantos *et al.* (1989) reported post-mortem survey findings that 90 per cent of patients reviewed had cerebral abnormalities. Table 5 summarises some of the more common neurological conditions associated with HIV disease.

Some problems associated with advanced HIV disease present management and symptom control issues. These include the following:

- vacuolar myelopathy (HIV)
- polyradiculopathies (CMV, HZ)

- distal symmetrical peripheral neuropathy (HIV)
- HIV encephalopathy.

Vacuolar myelopathy

This is thought to be due to HIV and presents with progressive ataxia, loss of power in legs and incontinence. Other causes of similar problems should have been excluded; the patient requires supportive care and physiotherapy to maintain balance and mobility for as long as possible or encouragement, when appropriate, to use a wheelchair and to maintain as much independence as possible. Some patients also develop myoclonic spasms, which may be painful. Clonazepam 1–2 mg bd has been found to be effective in some of these patients, but sedation may become a problem.

Polyradiculopathies

Cytomegalovirus has been found to be associated with a rapidly progressive syndrome of lumbosacral polyradiculopathy in 1 per cent of AIDS patients. They present with low back pain, sphincter disturbance and a progressive flaccid paraparesis (Fuller, 1992). CMV has consistently been found in the lumbosacral roots and treatment with ganciclovir or foscarnet may give improvement and prolong life in some cases. Herpes zoster has also been implicated in some. When treatment does not give improvement, supportive counselling, symptom control, bladder care and physiotherapy are all necessary to maintain quality of life for as long as possible.

Distal symmetrical peripheral neuropathy

This may be *non-painful*, presenting with altered sensation and numbness in toes or fingers, or a *painful peripheral neuropathy* which is sometimes very disabling. The painful variety is associated with axonal atrophy (Fuller et al., 1990) and presents with tingling, pins and needles, hyperaesthesia and shooting pains. Some have a burning sensation that is very unpleasant. Walking may be very painful or at least unpleasant, and some patients become more and more disabled and immobile as a result.

Patients with the *burning sensation* may respond to treatment with amitriptyline 25 mg bd or tds, or one of the other tricyclic antidepressants. Response to treatment is usual within 2–3 days and larger doses would make little difference. In some patients a non-steroidal anti-inflammatory agent such as diclofenac 50 mg tds will be effective.

Table 6. HIV encephalopathy

Early signs	Short-term memory loss intermittent confusion loss of concentration changes in personality and behaviour
Progression of encephalopathy	Diffuse neurological signs ataxia tremor limb weaknesses loss of coordination
Advanced encephalopathy	Total dementia Incontinence Grand mal attacks

Patients with *tingling or shooting pains* or with hyperaesthesia will usually respond better to an anticonvulsant such as carbamazepine or sodium valproate. The starting dose of carbamazepine should be no more than 100 mg bd for 2–3 days, then the dose may be increased to 200 mg bd or tds. There will be some reduction in the pain even at the lower doses. It is necessary to start with a small dose to avoid drowsiness, dizziness and nausea, but after a couple of days, an incremental increase should cause no problems. 200–300 mg bd or tds is usually sufficient to achieve good symptom control within 7–10 days. Some patients will do better with a combination of a tricyclic anti-depressant and an anti-convulsant. Flecainide and mexilotine have also been used.

A small number of patients will also require morphine, although painful peripheral neuropathy is usually only partially opiate-responsive (see also under 'Persistent and recurring pain' and Table 11).

HIV encephalopathy

This syndrome, also known as AIDS dementia complex (ADC), is well documented in advanced HIV infection, both secondary to the immune suppression and to the direct effects of HIV infecting microglia. MRI or CT scanning will reveal, in most advanced cases, some brain atrophy, although the degree of atrophy does not always correspond with the clinical findings.

Early minor signs of HIV encephalopathy may present in a number of patients with symptomatic HIV disease, but there is considerable debate about the presence of neurophysiological changes in asymptomatic people (Catalan, 1993). Table 6 shows the stages of development, with early signs including short-term memory loss, intermittent confusion and behaviour or personality changes, progressing through to the signs of advanced encephalopathy with total dementia and dependency. There is good evidence that Zidovudine will delay its onset, and also that it will give some (temporary) improvement in patients who have developed signs of encephalopathy.

Management This is a frightening condition for the patient, who in the early stages is aware of the short-term memory loss and intermittent confusion. It is also very distressing for a partner or relatives and friends to watch the deterioration taking place in the person's cognitive function and personality. Psychiatric problems may also develop, with disinhibition, personality or behaviour changes, restlessness and anxiety and occasionally with an acute psychosis. It is important to enlist psychiatric help in elucidating the problems and in the management of the patient. Nurses with psychiatric training may be very helpful in managing such patients, who will require increasing supervision and patience on the carer's part. Appropriate accommodation may be very difficult to find for these patients. Carers need a great deal of sensitive support and practical help, with offers of respite care from time to time to give them a break from the constant attendance and anxiety.

Drugs It seems that many of these patients become especially sensitive to any drugs that affect the central nervous system. Small doses of any sedative drug may cause excessive drowsiness, and it is therefore necessary to proceed with caution, starting with small doses.

Anxiety and restlessness may require a tranquilliser but the benzodiazepines may increase confusion and disorientation, thus worsening the situation while causing drowsiness. For these patients a neuroleptic, such as chlorpromazine or thioridazine which is less sedative and causes fewer extrapyramidal problems, may be very effective.

In those who require morphine, smaller doses than usually recommended are necessary to start with. 2.5 mg 4-hourly, rising after 24-48 hours to 5 mg 4-hourly would be best as a starting point, then titrating upwards as necessary against the pain. A patient with dementia may not be able, verbally, to express or explain pain; restlessness, body movements and facial expression may convey much to the experienced and observant carer.

Kaposi's sarcoma (KS)

In the West 35 per cent of patients with AIDS are said to present with KS (Kaplan et al., 1988). KS is more common when transmission has been sexual, i.e. in homosexual patients in the West, and in many parts of

Table 7. Classification of Kaposi's sarcoma

Stage	Tumour	Problems
I	Cutaneous, locally indolent	No systemic symptoms Body image
II	Cutaneous, locally aggressive	No systemic symptoms Body image, sometimes pain
III	Generalised, mucocutaneous Lymph node involvement	Weight loss Fever (unrelated to infection), ulcerations, lymphoedema, pain
IV	Visceral – lungs, gastro-intestinal	As above, with dyspnoea, diarrhoea, dysphagia and pain

Africa, where a slow endemic form of KS existed but is now being superseded by the more aggressive HIV-related KS.

KS may be classified into four stages as shown in Table 7. The prognosis in stages III and IV is related to the presence or absence of systemic symptoms, total tumour burden and the degree of immuno-suppression. Radiotherapy and/or chemotherapy may prolong life considerably, even in stage IV when the prognosis would otherwise be a matter of months at most.

The purplish lesions of KS are so obvious to the observer that many patients suffer as a result of the effect on body image. Camouflage make-up can be very effective (make-up and information may be obtained in the UK from, for example, the British Red Cross – see Appendix 1), but some patients become very isolated as they socialise less and less if the KS is on the face, for example. Radiotherapy and chemotherapy may effectively reduce or even cause a lesion to disappear, and will also reduce obstruction caused by oesophageal KS or progression of lung KS. Vincristine or vinblastine with bleomycin have been shown to be effective and well tolerated by patients with AIDS; conventional chemotherapy regimes are not so well tolerated in these patients (Gompels *et al.,* 1992). Radiotherapy given to oral mucosa may cause mucositis and ulceration and should be used with caution.

In the *terminal phase*, with widely disseminated KS, the patients may suffer extensive lymphoedema of lower legs, genitals, trunk and face. There may also be ulceration or cracking, with exudation, of cutaneous lesions. Skilled nursing care of wounds, skin and pressure areas is essential to reduce smell and can add considerably to the patient's comfort. The touch and closeness of carers, professional or voluntary, will help to reduce the self-disgust many patients feel. Lymphoedema is often a difficult problem in these patients. Peri-orbital and facial oedema may be dramatically reduced by dexamethasone 8–12 mg daily for 2–3 days, reducing the dose gradually to 1–2 mg daily over a period of 10–14 days. Dexamethasone may also improve the patient's appetite and sense of well-being. Very gentle and skilled massage of lower limbs and elevation may also help; intermittent pressure is not usually tolerated. Patients may need to be nursed on special mattresses as the skin is sensitive and likely to break down with any pressure.

Dyspnoea may be a problem with pulmonary KS and its associated pleural effusions which may be temporarily relieved by drainage. Morphine is the mainstay of symptomatic treatment for dyspnoea as it reduces the sensation and drive to breathe. Occasionally, patients who become too drowsy on oral morphine respond to nebulised morphine. Diazepam may also help to reduce the anxiety associated with the feeling of breathlessness.

For the treatment of pain see later under 'Common symptoms and their control'.

Skin problems

Skin problems (see Table 8) are extremely common in AIDS. Kaposi's sarcoma (see above) affects the skin in a substantial number of people with AIDS. Viral skin infections, such as herpes simplex and herpes zoster (see p. 66), are common and bacterial and fungal infections and eczema and psoriasis frequently occur. Recurring skin problems maybe an early sign of HIV disease, but skin infections or other conditions are almost universal in advanced AIDS. Scabies should be borne in mind as a possible cause of any atypical rash (see below).

Dry skin is found in almost all patients with the advanced disease, but is particularly severe in those who have suffered a slowly progressive debilitating process with persistent diarrhoea and weight loss, maybe as a result of malabsorption. The skin may be itchy and flaking, and therefore more vulnerable to secondary infection. Regular daily applications of moisturising cream and emollients applied to the skin or added to the bath may help to reduce itching and prevent secondary infection.

Seborrhoeic dermatitis/eczema commonly appears as reddened, sometimes scaly or crusting patches between or around the eyebrows, nasolabial folds, and in the beard and scalp areas, particularly around the hairline. It is commonly associated with fungal or yeast infections, and is best treated with topical steroids and anti-fungal creams in combination (1 per cent hydrocortisone to face, stronger steroids elsewhere).

Table 8. Common skin problems (other than KS and herpes infections)

Condition	Cause	Treatment or comment
Dry skin	?Malnutrition due to persistent diarrhoea causing reduced tryglycerides	Control of diarrhoea, and nausea and vomiting; diet and appetite stimulants; emollients
Seborrhoeic dermatitis	Often associated with fungal or yeast infections	Topical steriods and antifungal creams, Selsun shampoo, Betnovate scalp lotion
Folliculitis (generalised pruritic eruption)	Often associated with fungal or yeast infections	Anti-histamines, Eurax (crotamiton) NB exclude scabies
Psoriasis	May appear for 1st time in HIV-+ve person	Salicyclic acid, coal tar, Dithranol and strong topical steroids
Molluscum contagiosum	Pox virus	Phenol or silver nitrate applications
Ringworm	Tinea	Fluconazole, itraconazole, griseofulvin and anti-fungal creams
Norwegian scabies or crusted scabies	Very high number of scabies mites in immunocompromised individual; delay in diagnosis	Gamma benzene hexachloride applications × 3 initially followed by weekly applications for several months; possible need for strong topical steroids to reduce skin reactions

Scalp problems may be improved with the use of, for example, Selsun or Nizoral shampoo plus Betnovate scalp lotion or Synalar gel.

Folliculitis is a generalised pruritic eruption and may occur together with seborrhoeic dermatitis. Folliculitis may have the same aetiology as seborrhoeic dermatitis but it responds less well to treatment as the pruritus may be very severe. Anti-histamines may help to reduce the pruritus and applications of Eurax (crotamiton) may be helpful. However, bear in mind the possibility of scabies.

Psoriasis may appear for the first time in a person with HIV disease. It should be treated with the usual preparations such as salicylic acid and coal tar, dithranol or strong topical steroids.

Molluscum contagiosum is caused by the pox virus. It is common on the face, but also appears elsewhere as small papules with a dimple in the centre, which may become unsightly, and also interfere with shaving in the male. They may be treated with careful application of phenol to the centre of the small papule using the tip of a sharpened orange stick. Silver nitrate may also be used but cryotherapy is the most effective treatment. However, lesions tend to recur.

Tinea infections are extremely common and more aggressive than in the non-immunocompromised person. They may occur anywhere on the skin as ringworm, between the toes or as an infection of the nails. In the terminally ill patient treatment of nail infections may not be appropriate as this requires long term treatment with griseofulvin for many months. Itraconazole or fluconazole are alternatives and may be useful in any fungal skin infection which has become extensive. Anti-fungal creams, with or without steroids, should be applied regularly, 2 or 3 times a day for 2 to 3 weeks, to the affected areas.

Scabies should be suspected when a patient presents with any atypical rash which has persisted, or when crusting or nodules are present. In an immunocompromised host scabies may develop into what is known as Norwegian or exaggerated, nodular or crusted scabies (Ran and Baird, 1986), which is very contagious because of the increased number of mites carried by each patient. In an immune competent host there are estimated to be under 50 female egg-laying mites, whereas in Norwegian scabies the number of such mites may multiply to over 2 million per patient. The diagnosis may be delayed because the rash is atypical or may mimic, for example, seborrhoeic dermatitis. A diagnosis should be made by looking for the mite in skin scrapings, or scrapings obtained from under the nails. *Treatment* is more difficult in an immunocompromised person as repeated applications of scabicide may be necessary to eradicate the infection. In ordinary scabies 90 per cent of live mites are usually eradicated by one application of gamma benzene hexachloride (Alexander, 1968); in Norwegian scabies it may be necessary to continue with repeated applications for up to 6 months. Repeated applications may result in an irritant reaction for which it is necessary to apply potent topical steroids as well as scabicide. As mentioned above, Norwegian scabies is extremely contagious, not least because of the enormous number of mites shed in the scale into bedding and furniture. Although the scabies mite is thought to have only a short survival time outside the human body, in one unit caring for people with AIDS, staff who had not been in contact with the infected patient, but had used the same furniture, or had stood by the bedside, became infected. Six members of staff and three other patients became infected before the source was identified and it took three months to eradicate the infection from the unit. All patients, their partners or carers, and the staff and their partners needed treatment with weekly applications, and all the furnishings, including carpets and easy chairs, had to be treated. It is advisable that a dermatological opinion and supervision is sought early if Norwegian scabies is suspected in a setting where immunocompromised patients may be at risk.

AIDS-related cancers

Kaposi's sarcoma is the cancer that occurs most commonly in HIV disease, and has already been discussed. Lymphomas form the largest other group of AIDS-related cancers. The commonest type to occur is the high grade B cell lymphoma which may be found in the CNS, bone marrow, gastro-intestinal tract, liver, heart, lymph nodes, and may be single or disseminated. An increased incidence of other tumours may also occur. One study which compared the clinical diagnoses made in life with the findings at autopsy found that many lymphomas had been missed during life (Monforte *et al.*, 1992). Thus 26 (10.4 per cent) out of 250 patients with AIDS were found to have a non-Hodgkin's lymphoma on autopsy, as compared with 16 (6.4 per cent) diagnosed in life. Similarly, 16 cerebral lymphomas were found on autopsy (6.4 per cent), as compared with seven (2.8 per cent) diagnosed in life. The *prognosis* for patients with cerebral lymphomas is generally very poor, only a matter of months, even with radiotherapy. Other lymphomas may respond well initially to chemotherapy or radiotherapy.

In 100 patients admitted consecutively to Mildmay, 28 had cancers; 20 had KS and eight had lymphomas, three of which were primary cerebral. As median survival times are lengthening with improved treatment, more patients are developing lymphomas and disseminated or visceral KS, together with other intractable problems (Peters *et al.*, 1991).

The *main problems* associated with advanced AIDS-related lymphomas depend on the site and the degree of immunosuppression. Cerebral lymphomas usually present with focal neurological signs or with confusion and should be differentiated from toxoplasmosis, PML, HIV encephalopathy or other causes of confusion. Biopsy is the only definitive diagnostic investigation and because of the poor prognosis and response to treatment, is not always done. A trial of treatment for toxoplasmosis is usually advised; clinical response to treatment and CT or MRI scans to monitor progress will give clues as to the diagnosis.

Symptom control problems and supportive care in the terminally ill patient relate to the neurological deficits and headache with vomiting in cerebral lymphomas; in others there may be weight loss, anorexia and pain (see below under 'Common symptoms and their control').

Common symptoms and their control

Many of the symptoms encountered in advanced AIDS are those that would be encountered in any terminal care situation. Table 9 illustrates some of the most commonly encountered symptoms in 100 consecutive admissions to a hospice unit. This section will not attempt to deal with every symptom in detail; nor will it seek to take the place of the excellent books that are available dealing with therapeutics in terminal cancer or other life threatening illnesses. Here the basic principles from which to work will be outlined, giving some useful guidelines to those who may not be so familiar with this approach to care.

Many symptoms are directly related to a treatable cause, even in the terminal care situation. For example, herpes simplex infections in the ano-rectal region cause severe pain on defaecation and tenesmus, often persisting long after defaecation. This pain is best treated with a course of acyclovir (400–800 mg 5 times daily for 5 days). Analgesia may also be necessary until the acyclovir has taken effect. The pain caused by an anal fissure, may be soothed with lignocaine ointment or gel, but healing of the fissure will only be possible when the anus is no longer subjected to either the stretching associated with the passing of hard stools, or the maceration associated with frequent loose stools or watery diarrhoea. The anorexia and soreness of the mouth associated with *Candida* infections are best treated by controlling, as far as possible, the infection. Nausea and vomiting are frequently side effects of one or more of the many drugs that the patients are taking; where possible it may make a considerable difference to rationalise the number of drugs, perhaps reducing the dosages and the number of drugs being taken, or altering the times at which the drugs are being taken.

When it is not possible to eradicate the cause it is usually possible to control the symptoms.

Pain

Many different pains are commonly encountered in AIDS, especially in advanced AIDS. It is important to identify the type, site, severity and persistence of the pain being described. Each pain should be clearly identified and, where possible, the patient should be asked to quantify the pain by placing it on, for example, a visual analogue scale from 0 to 10, where 0 equals no pain and 10 equals the worst pain ever felt. This scale can then be used to monitor the response to therapy.

Table 9. Common symptoms on admission (in order of frequency) N = 100

Symptom	No's (=%)	Comments
Pain		
Neuropathic pain	22	HIV-related; tingling, numbness, hyperaesthesia
Pressure sore pain	12	Pain related to direct pressure and inflammation
Visceral pain (chest/abdo)	10	Associated with KS, lymphoma, constipation
'Total body pain'*	9	Diffuse overwhelming distress
Headaches	8	Associated with raised ICP or encephalitis
Joint pains	7	HIV arthropathy, septic monarthritis × 1
Epigastric pain/retrosternal	7	Herpes, candida, NSAIDs, lymphoma
Myopathic	5	May be related to AZT
Ano-rectal	4	Herpes infection, anal fissure
Other common symptoms		
General debility/wt loss	61	Most patients in advanced AIDS
Anorexia	41	Often related to mood/depression
Confusion/dementia	29	Differential diagnosis important
Nausea/vomiting	21	Often drug induced or related to crypto sp. or other infection
Depression	20	Differentiate from grief/sadness
Skin problems		Other common problems include
Dry skin	19	viral, tinea, and bacterial infections
Seb. dermatitis	14	
Scabies	7	
Molluscum contagiosum	4	
Psoriasis	1	
Cough	19	Dry, persistent cough, dyspnoea, ?PCP
Diarrhoea	18	Some treatable causes: cryptosporidial difficult to control
Constipation	18	Opioid therapy – treat pro-actively
Dyspnoea	11	?PCP, ?anaemia, KS, TB or other infective cause
Paralysis	8	Associated with CVA, toxoplasmosis, PML or lymphoma, myelopathy
Patients admitted moribund	8	

Total body pain

Total body pain is a condition in which the patient is overwhelmed and distressed by pain in several sites, and may include spiritual anguish with no particular focus. Total body pain may be the patient's response to overwhelming emotional distress, but it should be taken extremely seriously and treated as an emergency. The physical effects are similar to those of someone 'going into shock'. Once the overwhelming nature of the pain or other distress compounding the pain has been dealt with effectively, it is then possible to identify and deal with the details. Assessment should be made thoroughly but as quickly as possible, and an appropriate analgesic such as diamorphine should be given at once, sub-cutaneously or intravenously where necessary, together with an anti-emetic such as cyclizine, haloperidol or methotrimeprazine which also have a sedative effect.

Persistent or recurring pain

Persistent or recurring pain requires preventative therapy, i.e. analgesics should be given regularly and prophylactically. 'As required' medication is irrational and inhumane in this situation.

Twycross and Lack (1990)

The aim is to titrate the dose of analgesic against the patient's pain, gradually increasing the dose until we obtain the maximum relief with the minimum interference.

Swerdlow and Ventafridda (1987)

Morphine

The analgesic staircase (see Figure 1) illustrates the process by which pain may be controlled according to severity and response to analgesics. The response to therapeutic intervention should be monitored on a frequent and regular basis (e.g. hourly or 2 hourly in severe pain, 4 hourly or daily as appropriate in less severe pain). Once the decision has been taken to start morphine (or diamorphine), this should be given orally every 4 hours (elixir, tablets or suppositories are also available). It is usually recommended that 10 mg be given as a starting dose, but this will depend on what analgesia the patient has already been taking, how effective it has been, and on the condition of the patient. In very severely debilitated and emaciated patients smaller starting doses, such as 2.5–5 mg, may be necessary as some patients appear to be particularly sensitive and may develop unacceptable nausea and vomiting or drowsiness. A regular antiemetic, such as prochlorperazine or haloperidol, should be given with the morphine. However, the aim should be to control the pain as quickly as possible, with as few side effects as possible. If the dose given has not controlled the pain by 80–90 per cent the next increment up the table should be given. A chart for the conversion between morphine and diamorphine is given in Table 10.

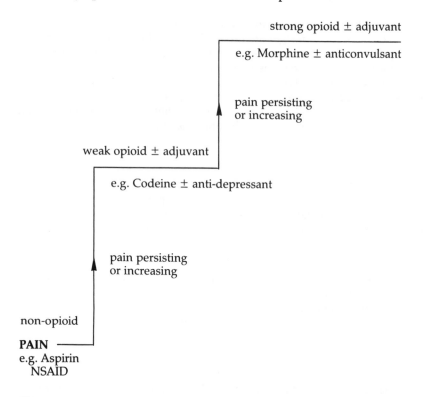

strong opioid ± adjuvant

e.g. Morphine ± anticonvulsant

pain persisting
or increasing

weak opioid ± adjuvant

e.g. Codeine ± anti-depressant

pain persisting
or increasing

non-opioid

PAIN
e.g. Aspirin
   NSAID

Figure 1   Analgesic staircase for persistent or recurrent pain. (Adapted from Swerdlow and Ventafridda, 1987.)

When pain control has been achieved and is being maintained on a 4 hourly regime it will be possible to change to sustained-release tablets of morphine sulphate (MST continuous) – these are taken 12 hourly and are therefore more convenient. The total dose taken over 24 hours should be divided by 2 to obtain the 12 hourly dose. (MST tablets are available as 10, 30, 60 and 100 mg.) (See also Table 10 for conversion to diamorphine, oral and injected forms). It is usually possible to stop the anti-emetic after a few days, unless other causes for nausea are present.

Adjuvants or co-analgesics

Some pains are resistant to opioids and respond better to combination with a co-analgesic or adjuvant drug. Table 11 shows the appropriate drug for the different types of pain. Rather than increasing the dose of opioid in the case of pain caused by the processes listed in Table 11, the

Table 10. Morphine and diamorphine conversion chart; 4-hourly dose equivalents

Oral morphine (mg)	Injected diamorphine (mg)	Oral diamorphine (mg)
5	2.5	2.5
10	5	7.5
20	7.5	15
30	10	20
45	15	30
60	20	40
90	30	60
120	45	90

Conversion ratios 3:1:2

Table 11. Adjuvants (co-analgesics) for some pain syndromes (adapted from Swerdlow and Ventafridda 1987)

Type of pain	Adjuvant or co-analgesic indicated
Inflammatory or bone pain	Aspirin or NSAID
Raised intracranial pressure	Dexamethasone
Nerve destruction pain (deafferentation)	Antidepressants or/and anticonvulsants
Intermittent stabbing pain (neuralgic)	Anticonvulsants
Gastritis/PU pain	Metoclopramide, cimetidine, ranitidine
Rectal/bladder spasm pain	Chlorpromazine, nifedipine
Muscle spasm pain	Diazepam, baclofen, clonazepam

addition of an appropriate co-analgesic drug may give much better pain control with fewer side effects. For example, in the case of inflammatory or bone pains the addition of a non-steroidal anti-inflammatory agent may achieve better relief than morphine. To reduce the number of tablets taken, and the side effects, the longer-acting forms should be used or those requiring only twice-daily dosages (e.g. sustained-release indomethacin, naproxen, ketoprofen or diclofenac). It may also be useful to prescribe these drugs in suppository form, although not all patients will accept these. Naproxen has recently been used in a syringe driver with good results (Toscarni et al., 1989).

The anti-convulsants carbamazepine or sodium valproate are particularly useful for the control of neuropathic, neuralgic or deafferentation pains.

Dexamethasone is effective for the relief of headaches of raised intra-cranial pressure, for which opioids are not very effective. It is useful, also, for its powerful anti-inflammatory effect, and will improve appetite and induce a general sense of well being. Dexamethasone will also reduce the facial and orbital oedema that may be caused by KS lesions. There are dangers of long-term steroid use and of masking infective or inflammatory processes, but in the terminal care situation these may be out-weighed by the aim to improve quality of life.

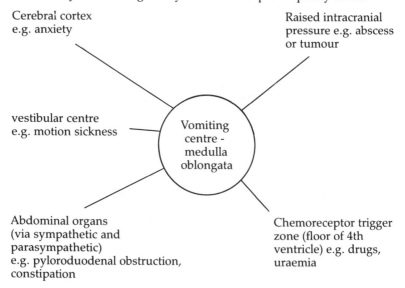

Figure 2   The likely causes of nausea and vomiting. (Adapted from Swerdlow and Ventafridda, 1987.)

Nausea and vomiting

Almost all patients with AIDS complain of nausea and vomiting at some stage, and for some it is extremely resistant to treatment. For many it is a transient problem but for some it is a continuing one, and contributes to anorexia and weight loss. It is important to diagnose the cause in order to prescribe the appropriate treatment. Figure 2 illustrates the likely causes – drug-induced nausea is the commonest, and that caused by, or associated with, cryptosporidial diarrhoea is probably the most difficult to control.

It may be possible to reduce or eliminate drug-induced nausea by rationalising the regime, simplifying it, or stopping certain drugs for a while. When other measures fail, adjusting the timing of drugs in relation to each other, or to meal-times, may be effective in reducing nausea and/or vomiting. Some drugs are available as suppositories and may be useful when the patient is vomiting, and/or objects to injections. The same rule applies to the treatment of nausea as to pain: it should be given regularly and not on a 'prn' basis, when it is persistent or recurrent in nature. Table 12 provides guidelines for the treatment of nausea and vomiting.

Intractable vomiting may be associated with, for example, cryptosporidial diarrhoea, or severe anxiety. A combination of antiemetics, working at different levels may achieve better control than a single drug. In some case it may be necessary to use a syringe driver to achieve good 24-hour control, and to enable a patient to eat and drink and to have some measure of quality. Once control has been achieved it may be possible to return to oral medication. Nabilone (1–2 mg po) may be effective where other treatments fail, but may cause euphoria or other CNS effects (Green et al., 1989) (see also p. 86).

Anorexia and weight loss

These very common problems may be treated with megestrol acetate (80–160 mg bd) which has been shown to increase weight as well as appetite (von Roenn et al., 1988). Periactin (4 mg bd or tds) may also stimulate the appetite, as will prednisolone or dexamethasone. However, in very advanced disease it may not be possible to achieve significant results for long, if at all.

Diarrhoea (See also 'Cryptosporidial and other diarrhoea')

Diarrhoea is a very common problem in patients with HIV disease. Where possible the cause should be identified and treated. Symptomatic treatment aims at reducing the number and frequency of stools, thickening the consistency where this would be helpful, and reducing colicky abdominal pain associated with diarrhoea. It is helpful to have a baseline from which to monitor response: i.e. number of stools in 24 hours, consistency (i.e. watery, soft, etc.). A bowel chart kept by the patient, perhaps with the help of a nurse, is a useful tool.

Rehydration may be necessary with oral rehydration solutions or intravenous fluid. Vomiting should be controlled, where possible, orally, by injection or via a syringe driver as necessary. If there is intractable vomiting and diarrhoea a syringe driver may be the most

Table 12. Treatment guidelines for nausea and vomiting (Recommended drugs are examples only.)

Cause	Drug: dose recommended	Comment	Site of action of drugs (main)
METABOLIC e.g. drug induced e.g. uraemia carcinomatosis	Cyclizine 25–50 mg tds**	EP effects	Chemoreceptor trigger zone
	Prochlorperazine 5–25 mg	Sedative/EP effects	
	Chlorpromazine 25–50 mg*	Sedative/EP effects	
	Domperidone 10–30 mg tds+	No EP effects	
	Metoclopramide 10–20 mg tds*	EP effects (60 kg or less)	
	Methotrimeprazine 25–50 mg tds*	Very sedative	
	Haloperidol 0.5–5 mg bd*	EP effects	
ABDOMINAL e.g. constipation gastritis	Metoclopramide 10–20 mg tds*	Promotes peristalsis and relaxes pylorus	Chemoreceptor trigger zone and local action
	Domperidone 10–30 mg tds+		
CORTICAL e.g. anxiety or psychological stimuli	Haloperidol 0.5–10 mg bd*	May cause EP effects at higher doses	Chemoreceptor trigger zone
	Prochlorperazine 5–25 mg tds*	sedative	
	Chlorpromazine 25–50 mg tds*		
VESTIBULAR e.g, motion sickness	Cyclizine 25–50 mg tds	Drowsiness, dry mouth	Vomiting centre
	Cinnarizine Dimenhydrinate 50–100 mg bd or tds		

Note: +does not cross blood-brain barrier
  * may be used in syringe driver
  ** tendency to crystallise in syringe driver
  EP=extrapyramidal

effective way to deliver both anti-emetic and anti-diarrhoeal drugs. Diamorphine and cyclizine or methotrimeprazine would be the drugs of choice for delivery through the syringe driver (see Tables 2 and 12). It is then usually possible to return to oral medication once control has been achieved. Equivalent doses of morphine sulphate as MST (sustained release preparation) twice daily will usually maintain control.

In less severe diarrhoea, loperamide is the anti-diarrhoeal of choice. It may be given in divided doses up to 32 mg over 24 hours with no significant side effects (O'Neill, 1992). The addition of ispaghula husk preparation (Fybogel) once or twice daily (Mulvenna and Moss, 1992) to thicken the stool, and sometimes an antispasmodic such as hyoscine butyl bromide (Buscopan) may help to reduce bowel activity and colic.

Codeine phosphate 30–60 mg bd–qds is another alternative, but side effects such as drowsiness or nausea caused by the opiate may be a problem. In end-stage disease the problem of addiction does not arise; quality of life issues are more important.

Constipation

Any patient who is taking opiates or other constipating drugs will experience constipation, and preventative action should be taken to avoid this common problem (except of course where the opiate is being used to control diarrhoea). Constipation can cause very severe colicky abdominal pain and nausea, or even vomiting.

Patients who are immobile, cachetic, and who have a reduced fluid or food intake are likely to become constipated. The contents of the bowel may not only require softening, but the bowel may also need to be stimulated. Encouraging fluid intake, attention to diet and mobilisation will help, but laxatives are usually necessary.

If there is a risk of constipation, start a prophylactic laxative such as codanthramer (mixed softening and stimulant activity) either as capsules or liquid (e.g. 1–3 caps nocte) or lactulose (softener) 10–20 ml daily or bd. Lactulose is very sweet and sickly, and may cause bloating and abdominal discomfort at high dosages.

Patients who are already constipated should be treated according to the severity of the problem. For example, glycerine suppositories (softening) or bisacodyl suppository (stimulant – must be in contact with rectal mucosa to act) may be sufficient to unblock the patient. If necessary, add an oral laxative such as codanthramer. Some patients will require enemas followed by carefully monitored oral laxatives. Again, a bowel chart may be helpful.

Typical requirements of patients on morphine (Regnard and Tempest, 1992)

10 mg morphine q4h : 2 co-danthrusate caps daily
30 mg morphine q4h : 4 co-danthrusate caps daily
90 mg morphine q4h : 6 co-danthrusate caps daily

Dyspnoea (See also Kaposi's sarcoma)

Dyspnoea is often caused by more than one factor, and the sensation itself causes increased anxiety and fear. The cause should, of course, be diagnosed and treated where possible, e.g. PCP or other chest infection. Cardiac failure may be treated with diuretics and digoxin as appropriate, anaemia with a blood transfusion. A pleural effusion may require thoracocentesis when this is appropriate – patients with extensive KS may not benefit greatly or for long and it would therefore normally be inappropriate in the terminal phase. The patient needs reassurance, company, and a cool draft of air from a fan or window. Relaxation therapy may be helpful.

Drugs

- *Diazepam*: 2–10 mg stat and bd or tds, to reduce anxiety.
- *Morphine*: start with small dose as for pain and titrate upwards to reduce respiratory drive. If the patient has already been taking morphine increase the dose by 50 per cent but monitor for drowsiness and nausea.
- *Nebulised morphine* may be useful in some patients who become too drowsy on oral morphine. Use 10 mg of morphine or 5 mg diamorphine initially.
- *Nebulised bupivacaine* 0.25 per cent (25 mg/100 ml) has an unpleasant taste so some patients will not find it acceptable.
- *Oxygen* may improve hypoxia and some patients find it psychologically reassuring.

The use of a syringe driver

The use of the syringe driver in terminal care is a well established practice. It is very useful as a tool for delivery of medication smoothly over 24 hours in order to

- achieve symptom control when the patient is no longer able to take oral medication
- control intractable vomiting and diarrhoea.

The medication is delivered sub-cutaneously through a 'butterfly' needle, the site of which should be changed whenever local skin reactions develop, which may be every few days, or once weekly. In those for whom skin reaction is a problem the addition of 1500 i.u. of hyalase to the syringe driver may reduce the reaction and prolong the time available at a particular site.

Drugs which have been found to be effective when using syringe drivers in the terminal care of patients with AIDS are given below.

Diamorphine More soluble than morphine, and used to control pain, diarrhoea and dyspnoea.

Hyoscine For reducing secretions in pneumonia or chest infections; also may help to control diarrhoea, and to reduce peristalsis in intestinal obstructions or severe colicky pain.

Methotrimeprazine Very effective anti-emetic, and sedative in terminal restlessness.

Cyclizine Effective, but has a tendency to crystallise in the needle or 'butterfly' tube unless well diluted.

Metoclopramide Effective and will mix with other commonly used drugs in the syringe driver.

Haloperidol Useful in anxious, agitated or psychotic patients, as well as to control drug induced emesis; will also mix with other drugs.

Chlorpromazine May be used for its sedative and anti-emetic properties.

Midazolam (Ainsbury and Dunfy, 1989). Useful for agitation and restlessness, or as an anti-convulsant in those who require one. Diazepam pr may also be used (4–8 hourly) to achieve similar control and will cause muscle relaxation (more effectively than midazolam) in someone with increased muscle tone, or in neck retraction.

Phenobarbitone May be used in a syringe driver but should not be mixed with other drugs.

The reader is referred to the reading list on p. 157 for further information about detailed symptom-control matters. In the care of someone with AIDS, as in any terminal care situation, it is the meticulous attention to detail, the degree of good communication between all concerned, and the teamwork, with compassion and understanding, which will make the ultimate difference to the quality of living and the dying, and the memories with which the patient's loved ones have to live in the years to follow.

Table 13 provides a summary of drugs which are used for the treatment of common problems associated with AIDS and HIV infection.

Table 13. Drugs commonly used for treatment of HIV/AIDS-related conditions

Drug	Used for	Doses	Side effects	Interactions
Zidovudine (Retrovir, AZT)	HIV or AIDS Inhibits replication of HIV virus	250 mg tds (various regimes, usually <1000 mg/24 h)	Myelosuppressive – anaemia with neutropenia, leucopenia, thrombocytopenia, nausea, vomiting, anorexia, abdominal pain, headaches, rashes and pruritus, fever, myalgia, insomnia, bluish nail pigmentation	Increased risk of toxicity with other nephrotoxic and myelosuppressive drugs. Probenecid increases plasma levels. Avoid chronic paracetamol use – increase toxicity. Caution with drugs that have hepatic glucuronidation
Dideoxyinosine (ddI)	HIV disease – as above	1 sachet bd (tablet form being developed) alternating with or alternative to AZT	Peripheral neuropathy, acute pancreatitis. Rarely, hypokalaemia and hyperglycaemia	Diuretics. Avoid alcohol and use with caution if h/o pancreatitis or with other drugs which may cause pancreatitis or peripheral neuropathy
Ganciclovir (DHPG)	CMV infections Acute	IV 5 mg/kg bd for 10–20 days	Bone marrow depression, neutropenia and thrombocytopenia, nausea and vomiting, eosinophilia, reversible LFT abnormalities, testicular atrophy, phlebitis	Other myelosuppressive drugs, e.g. zidovudine. Portable infusion systems for home treatment are available
	Maintenance	IV 5 mg/kg od 3–5 days/week		
Foscarnet (Foscavir)	CMV infections Acyclovir resistant HSV	Depends on creatinine clearance	Nephrotoxocity, anaemia, penile ulceration, nausea Hypo/hypercalcaemia, phlebitis, headaches	Nephrotoxicity and hypocalcaemia are more likely if concurrent pentamidine is given
Acyclovir (Zovirax)	Acute herpes simplex/zoster infections	400–800 mg po 5 × daily for 5–7 days (also IV) topl/cream	Rashes, GI disturbances, abnormal LFTs, renal impairment, neurological reactions	Probenecid increases plasma levels Ganciclovir also active against HSV, so acyclovir not necessary if g. is being administered
Dapsone	Acute PCP (combined with trimethoprim) or alone for prophylaxis	100 mg po/day (at least 2 h before drugs which increase gastric pH)	Nausea, vomiting, anaemia (NB.G6PD deficiency) methaemoglobinaemia, neuropathy, headache, agranulocytosis, hepatitis	Probenecid slows urinary excretion. ddI reduces absorption Nitrates and nitrofurantoin may increase the risk of haemolysis in G6PD deficiency

Drug	Indication	Dose	Side effects	Interactions
Pyremethamine	Toxoplasmosis	25 mg pyrimethamine daily (with dapsone 100 mg daily)	Rash, Stevens–Johnson syndrome, bone marrow depression, neutropenia, nausea, vomiting, abdominal pain	Folate antagonists may increase risk of haematological side effects. Folinic acid may be preventative
Pyrimeth + sulphadoxine (=Fansidar) or sulphadiazine	Toxoplasmosis	50–75 mg pyrimethamine od; 500 mg sulphadoxine qds or 1 g sulphadiazine qds		ddI may impair absorption Caution with other myelosuppresive drugs
Co-trimoxazole (Septrin)	Acute PCP	60 mg/kg IV bd or 480 mg × 8bd	Nausea, vomiting, fever, rash, leucopenia, thrombocytopenia, abnormal LFTs	Possible potentiation of hypoglycaemics, phenytoin, warfarin and methotrexate
	Prophylaxis	960 mg bd		
Pentamidine	Acute PCP	IV 4 mg/kg/day over at least 1 hour for 14 days	Hypotension (may be severe) Hypo or hyperglycaemia, phlebitis rash, nausea, vomiting, nephrotoxicity	Nephrotoxicity and hypocalcaemia, more likely with foscarnet
	Acute PCP	Nebulised 600 mg in 6 ml sterile water for 14 days	Bronchospasm (pre-treatment with β$_2$ agonist may reduce this)	
	Prophylaxis	Nebulised 300 mg in 3 ml sterile water every fortnight	As above	
Ketoconazole	Acute candidiasis Various mycoses	200 mg bd with food	Rashes, pruritus, GI disturbances gynaecomastia Few reports of fatal liver damage	Reduced absorption with high pH (antacids, H$_2$ antagonists), rifampicin increases metabolism. Enhanced anti-coagulation with warfarin and nicoumalone. Phenytoin levels enhanced in plasma. Ketoconazole absorption reduced by ddI.
	Prophylaxis	200 mg od with food		
Itraconazole	Acute candidiases Various mycoses	200 mg bd	Nausea, abdominal pain, dyspepsia and headaches	Antacids reduce absorption Rifampicin accelerates metabolism H$_2$ antagonists reduce absorption, also ddI
	Prophylaxis	100 mg od		
Fluconazole	Acute candidiasis Various mycoses	Up to 400 mg per day in divided doses	Nausea, abdominal discomfort, headache. Occasionally abnormal LFTs	Enhanced effect of phenytoin Nicoumalone and warfarin enhanced
Amphotericin lozenges	Oropharyngeal candidiasis	Up to 8 lozenges per day	Few except with IV administration	Increased risk of nephrotoxicity with aminoglycosides
Nystatin suspension/pastilles	Oral candida	1–5 ml qds 1 pastille qds	Nausea and vomiting in high doses	

Psychiatric problems

A wide range of psychiatric or mental health problems are associated with HIV infection although not necessarily caused by it. The 'worried well' are those who are not known to be infected but who are anxious, maybe even obsessively so, about the possibility of infection. The three main groups of disorders associated with HIV are psychosocial, psychotic and neuropsychiatric problems (Catalan, 1993).

Psychosocial problems

- Adjustment disorders
- Major depressive illnesses
- Anxiety disorders.

Those at greater risk include:

- Individuals lacking in social supports or experiencing major social problems, and those with a past history of psychiatric disturbances.
- Injecting drug users.
- Partners and relatives of those infected, especially in families where small children are infected.

Suicidal behaviour, including attempted suicide and deliberate self-harm, may occur in HIV infected people who may feel the situation to be hopeless, who blame themselves excessively, who see no meaning or purpose left in their lives, who have suffered personal bereavements or who may not be willing to become helpless and dependent. Counselling or psychological input is important, allowing the patient to express his feelings verbally or through art therapy. By expressing his feelings or having them accepted and taken seriously, he may find he no longer needs to act out his feelings.

Psychotic disorders

These include:

- Hypomania
- Schizophrenia-like illnesses.

These have an uncertain aetiology (Catalan, 1992) but experience at Mildmay would indicate that they are sometimes associated with episodes of very serious acute illness or with early HIV encephalopathy. Psychiatric support is important, and sometimes admission to a psychiatric unit may be necessary. For immediate control while awaiting help, give chlorpromazine 50–200 mg, depending on the problem or situation.

Neuropsychiatric problems

These may be related to complications of immune suppression and to the direct effects of HIV on the brain. HIV encephalopathy or dementia has been discussed earlier under 'Neurological problems'. In the early stages of dementia, personality changes and bizarre behaviour may develop which may include disinhibition about nakedness or sexual behaviour, extravagant spending sprees and grandiose ideas.

Management

Psychometric testing and psychiatric advice are helpful for differential diagnosis and management. Patients may require neuroleptics to control agitation but it should be remembered that they may be very sensitive and quickly develop extrapyramidal effects or become excessively drowsy on normal dosages. It is wiser to start with cautious doses and to use thioridazine or haloperidol, for example, rather than chlorpromazine or benzodiazepines. Sedative drugs may increase disorientation and confusion as well as sedation. A small dose of a tranquilliser such as diazepam may be helpful if anxiety is the main problem. The mainstay of care is in supervision and support offered, if possible, by nurses with experience in psychiatric or mental health work. A great deal of patience and compassion is required in caring both for the patient and for his/her family (see also p. 70).

References

Abonya, Y.L., Beamel, A., Lucas, S. *et al.* (1992). *Pneumocystis carinii* pneumonia: an uncommon cause of death in African patients with AIDS. *American Review of Respiratory Disease*, **145 (3)**, 617–20.

Ainsbury, B.D.W. and Dunfy, K.P. (1989). The use of sub cutaneous Midazolam in the home care setting. *Palliative Medicine*, **3**, 299–301.

Alexander, S. (1968). Clinical trial of a scabicide. *Medical World*, **106(7)**, 20–4.

Beck-Sague, C., Dooley, S.W., Hutton, M.D. *et al.* (1992). Hospital outbreak of multi drug-resistant *Mycobacterium tuberculosis* infections: factors in transmission to staff and HIV infected patients. *Journal of the American Medical Association*, **268(10)**, 1280–6.

Catalan, J. (1992). *Psychotic Illnesses in HIV Disease*. Abstracts of the Neurosciences of HIV International Meeting. Amsterdam.

Catalan, P. (1993). HIV infection and mental health care. WHO Second Report, Geneva.

Fitchenbaum, C.J., Ritchie, D.J., Powderly, W.G. (1993). Use of paromomycin for treatment of cryptosporidiosis in patients with AIDS. *Clinics in Infectious Diseases*, **16 (2)**, 298–300.

Fuller, G.N. (1992). Cytomegalovirus and the peripheral nervous system in AIDS *Journal of AIDS*, **5 (1)**, 533–6.

Fuller, G.N., Jacobs, J.M., Guiloff, R.J. (1990). Axonal atrophy in the painful peripheral neuropathy in AIDS. *Acta Neuropathos*, **81 (2)**, 198–203.

Gompels, M.M., Hill, A., Jenkins, P. *et al*. (1992). Kaposi's sarcoma in HIV infection treated with vincristine and bleomycin. *AIDS* **6**, 1175–80.

Green, S.T., Nathwarn, D., Goldberry, D.J. (1989). Nabilone as effective therapy for intractable nausea and vomiting in AIDS (Letter). *British Journal of Clinical Pharmacology*, **28(4)**, 494–5.

Kaplan, L.B. *et al*. (1988). Kaposi's sarcoma involving the lung in patients with the acquired immuno-deficiency syndrome. *Journal of Acquired Immuno-Deficiency Syndromes*, **1**.23–30.

Kovacs, J.A., *et al*. (1992). Efficacy of atovaquone in treatment of toxoplasmosis in patients with AIDS. *Lancet*, **340 (8820)**, 637–8.

Laine, L., Dresser, R.H., Conteas, C.N. *et al*. (1992). Fluconazole compared with ketoconazole for the treatment of candida oesophagitis in AIDS: a randomised trial. *Annals of Internal Medicine*, **117 (8)**, 655–60.

Lantos, P.L., McLaughlin, J.E., Scholtz, C.L. *et al*. (1989). Neuropathology of the brain in HIV infection. *Lancet*, **1(8633)**, 309.

Martin, M.A., Cox, P.H., Beck, K. *et al*. (1992). A comparison of three regimens in the prevention of PCP in HIV-infected patients. *Archives of Internal Medicine*, **152(3)**, 523–8.

Meunier-Carpentier, F. (1984). Chemoprophylaxis of fungal infection. *American Journal of Medicine*, **76**, 652–6.

Monforte, A.A., Vago, L., Lazzarin, A. *et al*. (1992). AIDS defining diseases in 250 HIV-infected patients: a comparative study of clinical and autopsy diagnoses. *AIDS*, **6**, 1159–64.

Mulvenna, P. and Moss, V.A. (1992). AIDS-related diarrhoea: a rational approach to symptomatic treatment. (letter.) *Palliative Medicine*, **6**, 260–61.

O'Neill, W.M. (1992). AIDS related diarrhoea: a rational approach to symptomatic treatment. *Palliative Medicine*, **6**, 61–4.

Peters, B.S., Beck, E.J., Coleman, D.G. *et al*. (1991). Changing disease patterns in patients with AIDS in a referral centre in the UK: the changing face of AIDS. *British Medical Journal*, **302**, 203–7.

Polis, M.A., Masur, H. (1989). Recent developments in the management of opportunistic infections. *Current Topics in AIDS*, **2**, 207–33.

Ran, R.C. and Baird, I.M. (1986). Crusted scabies in HIV infection. *Journal of American Academy of Dermatology*, **15**, 1050–9.

Regnard, C.F., Tempest, S. (1992). *A guide to Symptom Relief in Advanced Cancer*. Haigh & Hochland Ltd., Manchester.

Slavin, M.A., Hoy, J.F., Stewart, K. *et al*. (1992). Oral dapsone versus nebulised pentamidine for PCP prophylaxis: an open randomised prospective trial to assess efficacy and haematological toxicity. *AIDS*, **6(10)**, 1169–74.

Swerdlow, M. and Ventafridda, V. (Eds) (1987). *Cancer Pain*. MTP Press Ltd, Lancaster, UK.

Toscarni, F., Barosi, K., Scazzini, M. (1989). Sodium naproxen: Continuous sub cutaneous infusion in neoplastic pain control. *Palliative Medicine*, **3**, 207–11.

Twycross, R. and Lack, S. (1990). *Therapeutics in Terminal Cancer*, second edition. Churchill Livingstone, Edinburgh.

von Roenn, J.H. *et al*. (1988). Megestrol acetate for treatment of cachexia associated with human immuno-deficiency virus infection. *Annals of Internal Medicine*, **109**, 840–1.

Youle, M., Farthing, C., Clarbour, J. and Wade, P. (1988). *AIDS: Therapeutics in HIV Disease*. Churchill Livingstone, Edinburgh.

7

Counselling

What is counselling in the setting of terminal care for people with AIDS? In this situation counselling is the facilitation of a personal understanding of, adjustment to, and acceptance of the disease and its effect upon their lives, by the patients, the people important to them, and those caring for them. It is not the intention in this chapter to discuss how to counsel, but rather to highlight the particular needs and problems when caring for a person who is terminally ill with AIDS. Whilst most of the issues involved will be issues confronting any person with a life-threatening illness, there are differences which must be recognised and not underestimated. Despite attempts to educate and enlighten at national and local levels there still exists much fear and ignorance about AIDS and its transmission, even among health care professionals. This affects and often isolates patients and their families. Another difference was described very succinctly by Dr David Miller.

> In the West AIDS is associated with traditionally marginalised and oppressed social groups, subject to prejudice and cultural and legal oppression. Often our patients, as members of society, will have internalised many of those prejudices and those negative social attitudes about them, and so a diagnosis of AIDS will act as a catalyst for the expression of that internalised prejudice. It will result in a heightened potential for self destruction, whether it be in the form of an active response such as suicide, or a more passive response, such as self destructive guilt self hate or self pity.
>
> (David Miller, personal communication)

People with AIDS and their families live in constant uncertainty as to how and when the virus will affect them next and whether they will be able to cope. They also live with the perceived certainty that a diagnosis of AIDS equals death. Uncertainty may prove very difficult for many patients living with HIV antibody-positive status, fearing every cough and cold and wondering when and if AIDS will be diagnosed. It may be a relief when the person knows that they have AIDS rather than living with uncertainty.

Counselling should be available at all stages of this illness, from pre-screening counselling to bereavement support and counselling. The input to psychological and emotional care and support of people with AIDS and their families is often enormous, and clearly cannot always be given by fully qualified counsellors or psychologists. Staff of other disciplines within the team will often be engaged in activities relating to counselling, and it is important that opportunities are given to these staff to increase their knowledge and skills related to listening and counselling. It is essential, however, that team members, even those skilled at counselling, know when to refer patients on to the counsellor or psychologist, who can concentrate entirely on the psychological and emotional needs of the patients and those close to them.

The emotional needs of these terminally ill patients must be responded to wherever they are being cared for. Whilst in a few hospitals and community services, statutory service provision is made to help meet these needs, in others very little help is available. If patients are being cared for at home most of their help will come from the primary care team or from voluntary organisations offering support and counselling help. In some areas specialised home care teams are available and, as part of their remit, they offer emotional support and help.

In order to identify the feelings people with AIDS may commonly deal with, consider the factors that will create and/or influence those feelings:

- the shock of facing their mortality
- despair and hopelessness relating to the absence of a cure
- anxiety about the implications for family and friends
- grief relating to present and anticipated losses
- fear of the mode of dying
- anger at having been given infected blood or blood products, and/or at being the unlucky one, being caught out
- guilt; have I infected others?
- loss of self esteem and feelings of uselessness
- social isolation; real or perceived.

Whatever their coping mechanisms, people with AIDS are likely to be experiencing much grief. The Oxford English Dictionary describes grief as 'deep sadness'. In these circumstances the deep sadness of a person with AIDS is very understandable.

Peter is a young boy with haemophilia who now has AIDS. He is familiar with hospitals, having had repeated hospital admissions and is familiar with pain and disability. He has been excluded from certain activities and sports all of his life and, after repeated haemorrhages into his joints, he can now only walk with difficulty. Peter and his family have lived, and coped quite well, with fear, uncertainty and losses up to now. Now at 16 years of age he is dying. He has AIDS and the fears, social isolation and pain, both physical and emotional, associated with AIDS are touching him and his family. Peter and his parents are only able to share the diagnosis with a few key people, mainly those involved with his health and education. His parents have had to give him a lot of their time and feel guilty about his brother James. His mother describes the deep sadness she feels that, at only 19 years of age, James left home because of his own increasing isolation and pain as Peter became more ill.

Stress, grief and separation are putting pressure on the marriage. The parents describe it as 'rocky'.

Tracey has AIDS. She is now 19 years old but looks much older. Tracey used to live in squalor with her mother and two older brothers in a large council estate in Edinburgh.

When she was twelve, in common with most of her school friends on the state, she became involved in solvent abuse; 'We all did it, it was better than nothing, and there was nothing to do.' From there she went on to experiment with drugs and finally, at sixteen, she became addicted to heroin and shared 'works' with her friends. In order to finance her drug habit she became a prostitute, and stole goods and money from wherever she could, including her home.

Tracey's relationship with her mother became more and more impossible as her life-style became more chaotic and eventually, as she put it, 'Mum chucked me out'.

Tracey came to London when she was seventeen: with no money and no friends. She was given a home by a man who promised her food, and money to finance her drugs which she earned by giving her 'services' to him and to his clients. When Tracey became ill and was found to have AIDS she was again 'chucked out' and became homeless. After treatment in hospital Tracey registered at a drug dependency unit and is now taking reducing doses of methadone. She is self caring, but suffers from chronic tiredness and diarrhoea, and is living on her own in bed and breakfast accommodation. Tracey misses her mother and her friends but feels that she cannot go back now that she has AIDS.

Chris is 25 years old. He is a gay man and he has AIDS. For as long as he can remember he has felt different from other boys but he kept these feelings to himself and worried a lot. At 16 years of age he discussed these feelings with the family doctor who told him not to worry, he would 'grow out of it'.

Chris's parents had separated when he was fourteen and he had lived with his mother who was a teacher, and a strict Roman Catholic. He wanted so much to be 'normal', but finally decided he must accept himself as he was. Chris felt very sad about this as he loved children and wanted to be married and have a family, and now felt his homosexuality would deny him this. At the age of 20 Chris decided to talk with his mother about his situation. Her response was to cry, to hurl abuse at him and to distance herself from him. There had been a lot of press coverage about AIDS and it worried her. She decided that, despite the fact that he told her that he did not have a 'relationship' with anyone, he must have his own cutlery, crockery and towels etc. Every time he took a bath or went to the toilet his mother would clean the area with neat bleach.

Chris was a gentle, sensitive boy and it grieved him deeply that the one person he loved most in the world should reject him. He felt that God had rejected him too. Eventually his mother asked him to leave the home and Chris went to live with his father and his father's new wife. They allowed him to stay, but made him feel uncomfortable with their unkind comments and eventually, having got a good job, Chris rented a flat of his own. Rejected by society and by his own family he sought relationships that would be meaningful and fulfilling. After a series of disastrous relationships Chris met Martin who was also 21 years of age. They set up home together. The following 18 months were the happiest Chris had known. He was loved and cared for and about and felt secure in that love. Suddenly Chris became ill – he had diarrhoea and lost a lot of weight. He had been feeling tired lately and seemed to have no energy. Chris then got pneumonia and his worst fears were realised. He had AIDS; had he infected Martin? Martin was devastated. Here they were on the brink of life together with so much promise and it was all coming to an end. Chris wrote to his mother, but the letter was returned unopened.

Looking at these scenarios should enable the carer to see the other issues that many people with AIDS will need to work through, including

- child abuse
- separation
- rejection
- isolation
- disability
- drug and alcohol abuse
- loss.

The role of the counsellor

Whilst it is important that counselling should be available, not all patients will need, or wish, to use the service, and although the patient or client may have many problems, they cannot all be dealt with at once. The patient will indicate where he wants to start by introducing issues that he is ready to face and the counsellor must proceed only at this pace. Patients need time to help them face their losses and start the grieving process. Sigmund Freud talked about grief work – the idea of grief as a job of work which needs to be done if a person is to come through and get on with his or her life. Dr Colin Murray Parkes (personal communication) put it another way: 'It is a process of re-learning, it's a way of facing and coping with the new world which we are now entering, however much we may be reluctant to enter that world'. The role of the counsellor in this context, therefore, is to facilitate that re-learning and to help patients and their loved ones through the process of facing and coping with grief and loss.

Coping mechanisms may commonly be manifested in denial and anger. People with AIDS may move in and out of denial, only sometimes feeling able to attempt to face reality. Anger presents in many ways and can affect all the patients' relationships. He may be looking for someone or something to blame and anyone will do. Anger can be disruptive and cause much pain and hurt to the people who matter most to the patient. If a patient is able to see that, in this situation, anger is understandable and is part of grieving, he will be better able to deal with it. Most patients appreciate having someone who wants to listen to them, someone who is interested in what they have to say, someone who has the time. Some, however, may find talking very difficult, or be depressed and/or withdrawn. For these people it is important just to 'be there', keeping the care on offer and ensuring that they have access to the carer. Patients who have experienced social and emotional deprivation and have a poor self image may need more help in coping with their grief. Counsellors who anticipate the problems that they are going to meet, and the situations they are likely to confront, are likely to be better prepared when they do meet these situations. The person who is terminally ill with AIDS will also be better able to cope when he has had opportunities to discuss with a counsellor the anticipated problems or fears.

The counsellor should have considerable input to the care of those who are close to the patient. Family therapy, involving several members of the same family, is often needed. Lack of understanding and intolerance, long standing conflicts and separations and collusion between family members will often prevent the family from supporting the patient and each other. The complexity of relationships amongst the patients, may mean that those who are close to the patient will have many emotional problems. Specific problems with which the counsellor may be faced include the following:

- Male patients may have an ex-wife, young children, parents, a partner and an ex-partner, all of whom he may care about, and the counsellor may need to be involved with all of these people.
- Parents, who may be elderly and/or disabled themselves, sometimes for the first time facing the fact that their son is gay, are now also confronted with the fact that he is dying.
- Parents, still young themselves, and brothers and sisters are re-united after several years with their daughter/son or sister/brother who is now terminally ill.
- Partners of patients, who may themselves be HIV antibody-positive, watching the effect of the disease on the one they love. They have often had other close friends who have died and may still be grieving for them. Patients may have lived with their partner for many years and have had little contact with their family. At this time patients will often be re-united with their families; however the partner may be rejected by the family. The counsellor should be in a position to help the individuals concerned to deal with their conflict and bring harmony to the situation, although this is not always possible, usually because the parents/siblings are unwilling or unable to accept the partner. It is important to ensure that the wishes of the patient are respected and, if in hospital or a hospice, to arrange for separate visiting times for the partner and the family if necessary.

- Families of people with AIDS are seldom able to talk freely about their son's/daughter's illness and/or death in their own home town, hence may become isolated from friends and their support.
- Women with children who are HIV-positive may be overwhelmed by a sense of personal guilt: 'I have infected my own child'; or by anger directed at the partner who infected them both.
- As it is very difficult to identify the terminal stage of AIDS patients and their families may need counselling to help adjust to situations where apparent imminent death gives place to recovery.

Bereavement support and follow-up

Whenever possible bereavement support should begin before the patient dies. As stated earlier, if people are prepared for events they are much more likely to be able to cope with them. The families and friends of many people with AIDS have very little social support available. Gay organisations have set up support networks for gay men who are HIV antibody positive; this work has developed and now also offers support to heterosexual men and women. The value of group support cannot be underestimated. Organisations offering help include the following:

- Cruse
- Positive Partners
- BAHN (Black AIDS and HIV Network)
- Mainliners
- Body Positive
- Positively Women
- Terrence Higgins Trust
- London Lighthouse
- Mildmay Mission Hospital (see Appendix 1).

Memorial services and social evenings for relatives and friends of people who have died, and support groups for partners can assist in this bereavement process. Trained bereavement support volunteers, visiting people at home and referring back to counsellors if further input is needed, may also be of value.

Identifying the grief and loss people with AIDS and those close to them may experience can be a painful process in itself. The reader could be forgiven for thinking that being involved in the terminal care of people with AIDS is a thoroughly unhappy and depressing arena of care to be in – it is not. People with AIDS often have amazing courage and determination. Most are fighters – fighting for life. They do not sit around with counsellors 'coming to terms' with things; instead they are concerned with living. They are caring for, and about, those they love, caring about each other, and giving the carer the privilege of sharing in their lives.

A patient had just finished drawing a rainbow.
'There's one thing missing, though,' he said.
'And what's that?' asked the counsellor.
'A crock of gold.'
'What would you do with the crock of gold?'
'I'd spend it.'
'And what would you spend it on?'
'Life.'

Acknowledgements

Acknowledgement is made to the lectures on 'Bereavement and loss' given by Dr Colin Murray Parkes; and that on 'Counselling' given by Dr David Miller at the conference 'Terminal care for AIDS patients: an Holistic Approach' held in January 1988 at the Mildmay Mission Hospital.

8

Spiritual and pastoral care

'Even though I walk through the valley of the shadow of death, I
will fear no evil, for you are with me . . . '

Psalm 23

In providing for the care of the whole person the importance of spiritual
and pastoral needs must be recognised. Even the person who has no
faith in a God, and is quite content in his or her atheism, has a world
view, a system of beliefs about the world, its social systems, and his or
her place in them. A person's world view and belief system has a
profound effect on the way in which he or she faces issues of physical
illness, death and dying. Facing death can also challenge deeply and
long-held beliefs as nothing else can. It is then of the greatest
importance that there are people available to share that challenge, to
listen while he or she struggles with the often unanswerable questions
of life, such as 'Why me?' The question: 'If there is a loving God why
does he allow me, his child, to suffer like this?' may be asked. Usually,
the answer can only be 'I don't know'. Christians may share the convic-
tion that God suffers with the patient and that He wants to be there to
help carry the pain, seeing God's answers in the Cross and the Resurrec-
tion, giving hope. The words, however, will only become reality
through the carers actions, their presence, acceptance and sharing of
the pain. This is where faith without works is indeed dead, and will
mean nothing to the person who is suffering unless it is backed up by
practical action.

The person with AIDS may be facing particular spiritual conflicts and
emotional pain as a result of condemnation and rejection throughout
their lives. This condemnation and rejection may have been expressed
by the churches or the religious communities in which they have grown
up. Society's fear of AIDS has meant that people with AIDS are often
extremely isolated. This is true for all who are affected by AIDS. The
parent whose child is dying with AIDS may, with good reason, fear the
results of telling their neighbours or even their church fellowship or

friends what the real problem is. Elderly parents have been known to tell their neighbours and friends that their son was dying from cancer because this would at least ensure them sympathy. The single mother with AIDS who has one or two children, struggles alone for fear of her children being taken into care and the reaction of neighbours should it become known that she has AIDS and that her children may be HIV positive. Sadly, some Christians have only compounded the sense of isolation by their attitude and their preoccupation with judgement and theological discussion about innocence and guilt, right and wrong. The person with AIDS, therefore, is particularly vulnerable and sensitive, and may be afraid to speak or acknowledge spiritual needs.

As well as the fear that many people have of acknowledging and talking about spiritual issues, many will also have a deep sense of anger; anger at their God, anger at their particular religious community, represented by, for example, ministers of religion or chaplains. This anger may have to be expressed and accepted before any useful work can begin.

It is important that the multiprofessional team acknowledges that a person who is facing death has spiritual issues that need to be dealt with, and makes provision for these needs to be met. The person who is dying will choose with whom he speaks about such matters; it may be the home help, it may be the nurse or the doctor. It will certainly not be with anyone from whom he fears ridicule or condemnation and he may well be afraid of speaking with a chaplain or recognised minister of religion. It is therefore important that the spiritual counsellors or ministers of religion to whom a person may be referred are known to be sympathetic and understanding of the issues involved.

The hospice movement has done much to increase our understanding of the spiritual needs of people facing death. Several excellent books which deal with these issues in general, or in particular, are available (see 'Further reading') and provide a deeper coverage of the subject than is possible in this chapter. This chapter considers the *practice of spiritual and pastoral care* for someone who is living with AIDS and has to face issues of death and dying.

The carer must learn not to make assumptions or to use jargon.

A young woman had had little apparent experience of security, love or beauty. She said that she did not believe in God, but expressed fear of death, of hell and the afterlife. The concept of a loving father meant nothing to her, for in her experience the word 'father' was associated with abuse and neglect. It took time and patience to build up trust before any of these issues could be approached and then only on a very simple basis.

Theological discussion would have lost her completely. What she needed and wanted was love expressed in practical care, someone to sit and hold her hand in the dark when she was afraid at night to go to sleep, to read Psalm 23 to her when she wanted it, at her request to pray simply for God's acceptance of her, and to prove it by our continuing acceptance of her. This involved the whole team, and the people she chose particularly to talk with were those older members of the team who could represent to her a mother figure. The chaplain, too, played an important role in pastoral care and in planning with her her funeral and then taking it from Mildmay. She wanted Psalm 23 to be read at her funeral, and for all of us who were able to attend it left an indelible memory.

The role of the minister of religion in the multiprofessional team

For ease of reference the minister of religion or spiritual counsellor will be referred to as the chaplain. In a hospice the chaplain may be residential and a full member of the multiprofessional team, attending team meetings and being available to patients, their families and to staff on a regular and daily basis. Alternatively, hospices and hospitals may work with the local clergy and visiting chaplains, with ministers of religion from a variety of denominations or religions on call when required. In the community it is useful for the primary care teams to build up good links and liaison with the local clergy with whom they can work and to whom they can refer people when appropriate. However, as mentioned previously, it is essential that the attitudes and understanding of the chaplains or the clergy likely to be involved are fully understood.

The role of the chaplain includes providing for the religious needs (sacramental, ceremonial and ritual) that people have at this time, arranging funeral services, providing support and pastoral care for the patients, their families, partners and friends, liaising with other chaplains, ministers of religion and spiritual counsellors where appropriate, and last but not least, in just being there and available as a friend and supporter when needed and wanted.

Sacraments and rituals

Sacraments and rituals vary from religion to religion and from denomination to denomination, and may assume a greater meaning than ever before to someone who is living with AIDS and facing issues of death and dying. They may reinforce a sense of security and belonging and provide the means for expressing deeply felt beliefs without the need for discussion or exploration; they may serve, also, as a trigger to further discussion and exploration. Within the Christian tradition there may be the need for communion, confession and absolution administered by a priest; for some patients the services of Baptism and Confirmation will provide vehicles for establishing or re-establishing their sense of commitment to a system of beliefs; regular and special services may help and uplift; and for some anointing with oil and prayer for healing may be very important. Most religions have their own rituals and the chaplain may be needed to coordinate or facilitate these, bringing in the appropriate person to administer them at the patient's request. In many religions the last rites are of utmost importance and these must be respected by the people involved in providing care at this time.

Funeral services

As there may be some clergy and funeral directors who are unwilling to be involved in the funeral of someone who has died of AIDS, it is important to establish links early, discussing all issues at length and in depth. The funeral service should be conducted sensitively and with full understanding of the families/partners feelings and needs, including the full recognition of the partner's place in the person's life regardless of the legal status or general acceptance of that partnership. For many people living with AIDS, an important part of their positive approach is to think through and plan their funeral service, and the chaplain has an important role in facilitating this. Not all patients can do this however, and it is important for the families and partners to be able to turn to the chaplain knowing that he or she is familiar with their situations. Some patients may not wish to have a religious service. Some may want a celebration of their life instead of a funeral service and this may be a very moving and positive expression of their personality. There are now organisations that advise and help with secular funerals (see Appendix 1). Any rituals or ceremonies that are important to the person and those surrounding him should be given recognition through provision of time and space for these to take place.

Pastoral counselling and support

Pastoral counselling should be available to the person with AIDS, his family, partner and friends and others who may be important to him, and may provide a vehicle by which deeper spiritual care can be given. Pastoral counselling involves listening, sometimes counselling, often just being there and available. Sometimes it will take the form of very practical support such as providing company, taking someone for a drive, playing a game of Scrabble or chess. These activities may all form part of the 'bridge of friendship' over which deeper communication can take place and through which trust and understanding can be developed. It is possible to 'hide' behind the ceremonies or rituals, so as to avoid dealing with deeper spiritual or pastoral issues. Collusion between the chaplain, the patient and those close to him may enable the chaplain, as well as the patient, to avoid dealing with painful or difficult subjects. Ainsworth-Smith and Speck (1982), in their book *Letting Go*, identify four basic pastoral functions.

Reconciliation To facilitate a sense of reconciliation between the person and God, between him and those with whom he is in relationship, and within himself, with assurance of forgiveness.

Sustaining To support through personal presence and understanding, and through the administration of the sacraments, where appropriate.

Guidance To explain and/or guide the person through his exploration of belief and faith.

Growth To promote growth in maturity and wholeness.

Ainsworth-Smith and Speck feel that when time is short, as with someone who is facing imminent death, the focus should be on reconciliation and assurance. Pastoral support and counselling will facilitate this and may do much to promote the growth of faith and wholeness.

The attributes and needs of the pastoral carer

In providing spiritual care for terminally ill people with AIDS, chaplains, parish priests and/or ministers of religion should have sensitivity and wisdom, and have dealt, or be dealing, with such issues as sexuality, issues of death and dying, of loss and disability. They should have faced issues of sexuality within themselves and their own mortality. They should have an understanding and appreciation of their own ministry and pastoral identity, as well as of other religions, world views and belief systems. Pastoral carers should be aware of their own body language which may express their feelings on such subjects as homosexuality, guilt and innocence. Chaplains should understand and accept the anger, rejection and suspicion that they will often meet in those who feel themselves to have been rejected and condemned by their church or by their own religious communities, and often by their own families. Providers of pastoral care should be sincerely non-judgemental and accepting in their attitudes, and realise that the terminal care setting is not the arena for debates or statements on moral issues, but rather for comfort and strong reassurance.

Hospice and hospital chaplains, in particular, will need to have personal support as they themselves are facing conflict and questions which often arouse deep emotions. They may find their own strongly held beliefs challenged and their own identity threatened. They also will be facing multiple loss and bereavement having to conduct frequent funeral services for people who may have become friends. It is, therefore, important that the chaplain involved in this arena of care has a good personal support network and the support and understanding of the multiprofessional team.

The needs of staff and carers

Staff and carers involved in terminal care for people with AIDS will also be facing the same issues and challenges and may need pastoral support. They may need someone with whom they can discuss spiritual, ethical and moral issues. They may need someone to cry with and to pray with.

Thus the chaplain or minister of religion involved in the terminal care of someone with AIDS has a deeply challenging and vital role to play in the whole care of the person and all those who surround him.

Reference

Ainsworth-Smith, I, and Speck, P. (1982). *Letting Go.* Society for the Promotion of Christian Knowledge, London.

Further reading

See p. 156: Social, counselling and pastoral issues.

9

Practical issues related to death and dying

Much of the trauma and grief, and sometimes anger, that people feel at the time of bereavement, and which may be remembered vividly, often forever, is related to the practical issues surrounding death. It is important for all those involved in planning and setting up services for people with AIDS to have thought through, planned for and made policies relating to a number of practical issues. Some of these have been mentioned in other chapters but will be dealt with more fully here. Whilst many people with AIDS come from comfortable home situations and are surrounded by family and friends, some will be homeless, some will have no friends or family nearby, or with whom they have any contact, some will be living in squalid surroundings, and some may be single parents struggling to cope on their own with children who are perhaps also HIV positive or have AIDS. Wherever terminal care is being given, whether it be in a hospital, in a hospice or in the home, the following matters need thought and planning.

In preparation

Sorting out wills and other legal matters may weigh very heavily on someone who is facing their own imminent death. A member of the multiprofessional team, perhaps the social workers or counsellor, should ensure that there are appropriate forms available for those who wish to prepare their will, or to give power of attorney to a next of kin or other person of their choice. People with AIDS may require access to legal advice, but it is important to ensure that the solicitors involved are aware of and sympathetic about the issues related to AIDS. Serious family conflicts and traumas can be avoided if these matters are dealt with sensitively and properly by people who have experience in helping those who are affected by AIDS. Families may contest a will if property or substantial sums of money have been left to a partner or a charity of whom the family do not approve. Those involved in a patient's care, particularly if working for a charity or organisation which may have been a beneficiary of the will, should not act as witnesses to the signing of a will. The doctor may have to be involved in certifying that the patient is of sound mind while signing any legal document. In any such situation the doctor must be satisfied that the patient understands the implications of what he is doing, at the time at which he is doing it, even if his understanding is shortlived as in the case of someone who is suffering from intermittent confusion.

During the past few years the question of *living wills* has been hotly debated. Some see them as the 'thin end of the wedge' which might open the door to legalised euthanasia. Others feel they have a place if carefully worded and certain safeguards are instituted. A living will is a written statement made and signed by the patient about his wishes regarding active or emergency resuscitation if he becomes unable to speak for himself. Living wills are not as yet accorded legal status in Britain, but they are generally accepted as indicating the patient's wishes, giving guidelines when dilemmas are faced regarding the active prolongation of life in someone who has become severely ill, unconscious or demented.

In 1993 the Terrence Higgins Trust (THT) published and made generally available a form which may be used when making a living will. The implications of the choices being made by the patient must be fully explained to the patient by a doctor, who must be satisfied that the patient is of sound mind. The signature of the patient must be witnessed on the form signed by the witness. This form has proper safeguards written into it and makes clear and simple statements which may be readily understood. A pro-euthanasia organisation has also published a form; unfortunately this fact does confuse the issue and links living wills with euthanasia in many people's minds; a link which is, in the author's opinion, quite unnecessary and unhelpful.

An example of the questions and options available in the THT living will document is given in Figure 3 (p. 109).

Funeral arrangements

There may be many funeral directors, undertakers and staff at crematoria who are unwilling, through fear or ignorance, to deal with people with AIDS. The potential for distress to the partner, relatives or friends of patients will be reduced if the services of undertakers who have thought through the issues surrounding funeral arrangements for people with AIDS are used. Funeral directors may be able to advise as to which crematoria staff will deal sympathetically with the families and friends of those dying with AIDS. The families will often be extremely

Three possible health conditions are described below.

For each of the three, either choose A or B by ticking the appropriate box, or leave both boxes blank if you have no preference. The choice between A and B is exactly the same in each case.

Treat each case separately. You do not have to make the same choice for each one.

I DECLARE that my wishes concerning medical treatment are as follows:

CASE 1 – Physical Illness

If –
■ I have a physical illness from which there is no likelihood of recovery, *and*
■ it is so serious that my life is nearing its end:

A. I wish to be kept alive for as long as reasonably possible using whatever forms of medical treatment are available. ☐

B. I do not wish to be kept alive by medical treatment. I wish medical treatment to be limited to keeping me comfortable and free from pain. ☐

CASE 2 – Permanent Mental Impairment

If –
■ my mental functions become permanently impaired with no likelihood of improvement, *and*
■ the impairment is so severe that I do not understand what is happening to me, *and*
■ I have a physical illness:

A. I wish to be kept alive for as long as reasonably possible using whatever forms of medical treatment are available. ☐

B. I do not wish to be kept alive by medical treatment. I wish medical treatment to be limited to keeping me comfortable and free from pain. ☐

CASE 3 – Permanent Unconsciousness

If –
■ I become permanently unconscious with no likelihood of regaining consciousness:

A. I wish to be kept alive for as long as reasonably possible using whatever forms of medical treatment are available. ☐

B. I do not wish to be kept alive by medical treatment. I wish medical treatment to be limited to keeping me comfortable and free from pain. ☐

Figure 3 Part of the living will published by the Terrence Higgins Trust.

grateful and relieved to be able to take the advice of carers who have already set up good links with undertakers.

A young man died at home having been cared for effectively by the primary care team. The district nurse suggested a well known local firm of undertakers to the family who were then left to contact the undertaker. When the men came to remove the body and found out that the patient had died from AIDS, they refused point-blank to take the body.

Such distressing situations may be avoided by carers exploring which of the local undertakers are willing to deal with people with AIDS. Families of people with AIDS may be relieved to be able to take the advice of carers who have established good arrangements with particular undertakers.

The National Association of Funeral Directors has dealt with the issues surrounding AIDS and do have well thought out policies. However, not all funeral directors accept or follow these.

People who have been receiving income support, family credit or housing benefits may be entitled to assistance with funeral fees. The social worker or welfare assistant should be able to advise and help with arranging for this assistance. For patients who have died without funds of any sort it is possible to arrange a funeral through the local authority. Each local authority will have a contract with a particular undertaker and will use a specific crematorium so that there will be little choice. If a burial is wanted this may take place in a public grave which may hold up to eight adults. The funeral will take place at the discretion of the undertaker and will often, therefore, be in the early morning.

The transport of ashes or a body to another country may pose problems. Ashes being taken out in an urn will usually cause few problems and the undertaker will be able to advise. The funeral director or crematorium will have to supply a certificate of packaging and the death certificate should also be available. There may be different requirements for each country and a small fee may be payable. A container may be sent through the post, in which case a form of declaration has to be obtained from the crematorium and a customs declaration filled in. Again the funeral director will be able to advise.

Transporting a body from one country to another is likely to cause more problems, and the details should be explored and understood as far as possible before such a situation actually arises. It should be noted that limited resources and decreasing funds from charities may make it impossible to raise money for sending bodies abroad. The money may have to be raised by the family concerned. It is important to know, for example, that if the body of a Jewish person is to be flown to Israel this has to be arranged so that the body arrives in time for burial within 24 hours of death. Jewish undertakers will know the details and links should have been set up with a local firm. Problems are most likely to arise at a weekend and it is important to have some emergency numbers available. Each country will have its own requirements and the appropriate consulate or embassy will be able to give the details of what is required for their country. Two certificates are generally required, one to be issued by the doctor involved in the care of the patient which declares that the body is not infectious, and a second certificate issued by the District Medical Officer to certify that there are no significant infectious diseases in the district. Most countries also have strict specifications for the coffin which has to be zinc lined; the rules are not so stringent if the body is going to Ireland and a few other countries such as Nigeria. Italy has particularly stringent specifications and these increase the overall cost of transporting a body.

Viewing a body

When planning for terminal care in any hospital, hospice or sheltered accommodation it is important to plan for the viewing of a body after death, either in the patient's own room or in a separate room or small chapel of rest. Wherever viewing takes place it should be in quiet, dignified, and comfortable surroundings but where the body can be kept relatively cool for as long as possible. The body may be kept, with safety, in a cool environment for up to 12 hours (occasionally longer), enabling relatives and friends who have a distance to come to attend without undue pressure.

Body bags

In the United Kingdom guidelines specify that the body of someone who has died with AIDS should be placed in a body bag after death and not re-opened again. There does not appear to be any particular logical or scientific reason for this, and in many other countries there are no such rules. Nurses who encounter this for the first time may find it extremely distressing to have to do and, of course, it can be very distressing for relatives and friends of the patient whose body has to be placed in the body bag. The bags themselves are made from semi-opaque heavy duty plastic in various sizes with a zip, and may be obtained from commercial firms; it is important to know who is the local supplier.

The guidelines state that all bodies must be labelled 'Risk of infection' – the label should be placed discreetly, e.g. on the ankle, so that any family member who does not know the full diagnosis is not suddenly faced with the knowledge at a particularly bad time. However, it must be sufficiently clear so as to warn an undertaker who is not aware of the diagnosis and who may be asked to undertake embalming. The body bag, too, should be discreetly labelled 'Risk of infection'. It is also important to have thought through the policy of the multiprofessional team relating to the use of body bags. The body can be laid out as for any patient who has died, with viewing taking place before the body is wrapped in a sheet, placed into a body bag and removed by the undertakers. However, adherence to the Department of Health guidelines can cause difficulties in fulfilling other legal requirements. If the body is to be cremated it has to be seen by two independent doctors. The first doctor is the patient's usual medical practitioner or the doctor who has cared for him during his terminal illness; the second doctor should be independent, i.e. not working in the same practice or team; he or she has, by law, to examine the body before filling in the second half of the cremation form. This means that the doctor has to unzip the body bag and unwrap at least part of the sheet in order to be able to fulfil the law as it is not usually possible for the second doctor to be available immediately after death; the second examination may take place a day or two later at the undertakers. It makes good sense to use body bags when there is leakage of body fluids.

Accommodation for partners, family and friends

There are, as yet, very few hospices which will take people with AIDS; this may mean that those who do will of necessity have to take patients from a very wide catchment area. Hence, when planning for any institutional care of patients who are dying with AIDS, it is important to remember that many may have families who live a long way away, and that the families may have difficulty in finding accommodation at short notice. If possible, provision should be made to enable visitors to stay in or near the hospital, hospice, or wherever care is taking place. In planning accommodation it is also important to plan for support for the families or visitors who will be staying in that accommodation. It is extremely exhausting and draining for nurses who are caring for the patients to also be constantly supporting the relatives and friends of the dying patient. If no arrangements are made to enable relatives and friends to leave the ward or the unit and to find support through other team members, the full burden of their support falls onto the nursing staff, or sometimes even onto other patients and their visitors. This is, of course, not so in the home setting in the community. In this setting it may be helpful to make arrangements for relatives to meet with a counsellor, or with the doctor, or social worker in the health centre or in an office away from the home. It may be necessary to arrange for a volunteer or another member of the team to stay with the patient in order to give the family and carers a break, so that they themselves can go and find some relief or support outside the home and away from the patient.

When the patient is dying

In the final few days or weeks of a patient's life, it should be borne in mind by all, and at all times, that the overall aim of care is to enable the patient to die in comfort and dignity. There should be a continuing respect for the patient's wishes, even if he is unconscious. There should also be a respect for any religious requirements or needs that may have been expressed or which are implicit in the religion to which the patient belongs, for example, any last rites that are important to a Catholic, to a Jew or to a Muslim, or to a member of any other religious community. The person who has been caring for the patient could easily feel pushed out at this point by professionals who come in and take over, or by family members who may not, until then, have been much in evidence. The primary carer, if involvement is wanted, should continue to give whatever care he or she feels able to give, cooperating with the nurse as to who does what. In hospitals care is usually given by the nurses; in hospices and in the home setting the families or partners are more frequently involved in the actual care of the patient. It may be necessary for the nurse to perform certain procedures, and it may be better for the carer and for the patient if the direct carer is not too closely involved, particularly in some of the more distressing procedures, for example the dressing of a pressure sore or the giving of an enema.

As death approaches meticulous attention to detail is essential and communication between nurses and doctors in the monitoring of symptoms and responses to medication is of even greater importance than usual. It is important to plan for the provision of support and care for the family, partner, and friends as they grieve in anticipation and as they watch at the bedside. Plans should also be made to ensure that, if at all possible, the patient is not left alone at any time. A chaplain, priest or other religious leader, as appropriate, should be available both to the patient and to the family throughout, but a nurse or any other person may say a simple prayer of committal should this be wanted.

When the patient has died

Death must be ascertained and certified by a doctor, but when death has occurred there is no need to await the doctor's arrival before laying out the body. However, before beginning any such procedure it is important to ensure that the wishes of the family are known. Cultural and religious practices must be respected and provision should be made for those who need a place in which to mourn or sit with the body for a prescribed length of time, such as 24 or 48 hours as is required in some religions. Such a place should be relatively private and perhaps even soundproof as there may be chanting or wailing taking place which could disturb other patients.

If the family are happy to allow the nurses to wash and dress the patient and to lay him out, this should be done in the family's choice of clothes. It should, of course, be done taking full body fluid precautions as there may be some leakage of body fluids. Any person who lays out the body should be issued with gloves and aprons. For the purpose of viewing, the body should be made to look comfortable, with the arms outside the sheet. The body should be placed in the body bag after all the viewing has taken place. As mentioned in the previous section 'In preparation', policies regarding these matters should have been thought through and the details decided upon before the nurse and mourners are faced with this situation.

The mourners may wish to be alone with the body for a while although the nurse or other professional involved should offer to stay with them should they wish it. They may wish also to discuss suitable local undertakers although, as already suggested, this matter may be better discussed when preparing for the imminent death. The health care professional who has been involved should liaise with the undertaker on behalf of the family, and should also arrange with the family when they wish to collect the death certificate which will be issued by the doctor. This may be on the following day and the next of kin or another representative of the family should take the death certificate to the Registrar of Births and Deaths to register the death as soon as possible.

The doctor should take care as to the wording on the death certificate (see also p.51). It is likely to be extremely distressing for many families to see the words 'AIDS' spelt out. Where possible the wording on the certificate should be discussed with the family beforehand. Death certificates are not confidential documents, and are available for inspection by insurance companies etc. For correct statistical analysis and for planning purposes it is, of course, important that the cause of death is correctly reported, but the word AIDS should be avoided until health care professionals and society in general have stopped responding to the person with AIDS, or those who are linked to him, with fear, stigmatisation and discrimination.

It is important that those close to the person who has died are assured of continuing support and availability of the members of the caring team. The chaplain or minister of religion should be available for pastoral care and for discussion about funeral arrangements. The doctor should be available to the family, who may have questions or worries that they wish to discuss and there may be other practical matters to be dealt with. The interval between death and the funeral will be a fairly busy time with practical issues taking precedence over feelings. Bereavement support and follow up is very important at a later date and all those who are grieving should be reassured that this will be available to them when they need it. The health care professional should be aware that the bereaved person may need to express grief in tears, and should allow time and space for them to do so. Their need to express anger should also be accepted, remembering that the anger and sense of helplessness about the illness may well be displaced on to those who have been caring for the bereaved person's loved one. This anger should not be taken personally, although genuine cause for complaint should be investigated and dealt with. The whole team should be aware of and supportive of others throughout this time; one person should never be left alone to have to deal with several different groups of grieving people

The good memories that people take away with them from this situation will depend, to a great extent, on the sensitivity with which the nurse and the doctor and any other members of the team deal with the small matters and details. For some it may be a simple prayer of committal that is said by the nurse at the time of death which will stand out in their memory and bring comfort. For others it will be the memory of a peaceful face, of being able to hold his hand and having that physical contact for the last time. For others it will be the inclusion of a poem or a specially loved personal possession in the body bag before the body is taken away.

Some months after his partner's death, one man commented: 'The care that the team gave was very professional. They thought of everything. But what mattered most was the feeling of family which they created, the way in which we all shared in the caring and in the grieving.'

Reference

UK Health Departments (1990). *Guidance for Clinical Care Workers: Protection against Infection with HIV and Hepatitis Viruses. Recommendations of the Expert Advisory Group on AIDS.* HMSO, London.

10

Intravenous drug use and advanced HIV disease

Introduction

HIV is having a major impact on injecting drug users (IDU) throughout the world. The first known cases of AIDS in IDUs occurred in America, but there has been a rapid spread to many developed and developing countries The spread has followed the distribution routes of illicit drug trafficking (Des Jarlais *et al.* 1992) across s 'uthern Europe from Yugoslavia to Spain, across southern Asia fron southern China to northern India, and north to south in Brazil. A change from smoking, chewing or sniffing to intravenous use of highly refined, more compact forms of drugs such as heroin and cocaine has taken place. This may be related, in part, to the international and local police crackdown on the bulkier, less refined forms, and to the increasing availability of injectable, highly lucrative forms as countries become more sophisticated and industrialised. Table 14 shows the countries in which there is currently an increasing, or even a major IDU related epidemic.

Certain areas experienced a particularly rapid increase in the incidence of HIV among drug users. This appears to be associated particularly with an initial lack of awareness of HIV/AIDS, together with certain circumstances that facilitated rapid transmission among drug users (Des Jarlais *et al.*, 1992), e.g. the existence of 'shooting galleries' where injecting equipment is rented or shared and returned unsterilised to be used by other drug users. This occurred in Edinburgh in 1983–4 after a crackdown by the police on drugs and equipment. Bangkok, in Thailand, is another city where rapid spread took place during 1988, raising the seroprevalence from 2 per cent in 1987 to 16 per cent in the spring and 46 per cent in the autumn of 1988.

Following this increase the situation stabilised, largely through vigorous education campaigns, and in 1989, 92 per cent of IDUs

Table 14. Countries in which HIV infection among IV drug users is a serious problem (Des Jarlais et al., 1992)

Europe	
Austria	Poland
Belgium	Portugal
Denmark	Norway
Finland	San Marino
France	Spain
Germany	Sweden
Greece	Switzerland
Ireland	Turkey
Israel	UK
Italy	Yugoslavia
Luxembourg	

North America
  Canada
  United States
  Caribbean countries

South America
  Argentina
  Brazil

Asia
  China
  India
  Mayanmar (Burma)
  Thailand

Australia

reported that they had changed their behaviour to reduce risk of HIV transmission.

Other cities or areas with similar patterns of spread, leading to HIV seroprevalence rates among IDUs of above 40 per cent include New York, Milan in Italy, Paris in France and Manipur in India. Drug dealers sometimes lend equipment to customers for immediate use after buying the drug; in some cities drug users congregate in large groups near drug distribution centres, buying drugs and sharing the injecting equipment.

Patterns of spread may be related also to the drugs commonly available for IV use. Heroin has been the most commonly used drug (e.g. in Edinburgh, Bangkok and Manipur), but there are reports that cocaine in New York and in South America is associated with even greater risk of HIV spread (Lenkefeld, et al., 1990, pp. 120–31) as it is short-acting and some users will inject 10–15 times in one day. 'Speedballing' (mixing cocaine and heroin) will prolong the effects;

amphetamines, also CNS stimulants, are longer acting and this, among other factors, may lead to a lower risk in users who favour these drugs. Lower social status, conflicting relationships, homelessness and unemployment are generally associated with higher transmission and prevalence rates. This also means that the social and emotional supports that an ill person so much needs will often be lacking for an IV drug user with AIDS.

Clinical problems

Non-AIDS manifestations of HIV and drug use

Injecting drug users are subject to a number of problems and conditions that are due to factors such as the use of non-sterile equipment, a chaotic and stressful life-style in search of the next 'fix', and the frequently unhealthy environment in which many live. Those who are immunosuppressed as a result of HIV are even more likely to suffer recurrent skin infections, injection site abscesses and septicaemia. Bacterial pelvic inflammatory disease, cervical cancer and recurrent vaginal candidiasis are all common and very debilitating or potentially serious conditions in women. Tuberculosis may also be an ongoing and debilitating problem.

HIV is now considered to be the most important risk factor for tuberculosis in the United States. During 1990–92, 28,000 more cases of tuberculosis than were expected were diagnosed in the US – the precise role that HIV has played in this has not been determined as yet (Des Jarlais et al., 1992). Pulmonary tuberculosis is more common in IDUs than the atypical forms of mycobacterial disease. HIV is closely linked to increase in tuberculosis in Africa and Italy (Antonucci et al., 1992), and the same pattern is likely to emerge amongst infected IDUs in other parts of the developing world (see also Chapter 6). There is a high risk of active tuberculosis in immunocompromised HIV-infected IDU individuals (Selwyn et al., 1992). Staff who are involved in the care of an HIV-infected IDU patient with open tuberculosis should be Mantoux tested and, if necessary, vaccinated, and when appropriate should have chest X-rays and be followed up.

Hepatitis B is common among IDUs and 10 per cent of those who have had an episode become carriers. Staff caring for IDUs should be vaccinated against hepatitis B.

AIDS and HIV related conditions

A study of a large cohort of HIV infected patients being cared for in four hospitals in New York in 1989 found that IDUs were MORE likely to suffer from PCP, oesophageal candidiasis, extrapulmonary TB and bacterial pneumonias than patients with other risk factors. Drug users are LESS likely to have Kaposi's sarcoma, CMV disease, cryptosporidiosis and lymphoma than homosexual patients (Greenberg *et al.*, 1992). There is a markedly higher incidence of thrombocytopenia in HIV infected drug users. One study in Amsterdam showed that the incidence amongst HIV negative IDUs was 8.7 per cent whilst it was 36.9 per cent in those who were HIV positive. It was also significantly higher than in HIV positive individuals with other risk factors (Mientjes *et al.*, 1992). The higher prevalence appears to be related to a history of intravenous drug use, but not to recent injecting.

Care for IV drug users with advanced HIV disease

The main problems tend to centre around the following issues:

- chaotic life-style, unpredictable interaction with staff and/or other patients
- lack of support structures such as close family or friends
- the 'drive' to steal or prostitute to obtain drugs
- manipulative behaviour
- the needs of women IDUs with children
- financial problems
- homelessness
- continuing IV drug use on a regular or an intermittent and unpredictable basis
- methadone maintenance or a reducing programme?
- to stabilise or to 'come off'?
- symptom control and/or effective palliation or treatment in patients who are already 'loaded' with certain drugs such as opiates
- patients' knowledge of certain drugs.

Social problems and issues

The social issues form a background against which clinical care must be given, either in the home or in hospice or hospital settings. Many drug users started at a very early age, maybe as a result of poverty and a sense of hopelessness, maybe because everyone else in the street or on the estate was thought to be using drugs. The peer pressure, or the longing to belong, may make it very difficult for young children to stand out against drug use with the result that, by the time they become ill, they are already well into the life-style and are truly addicted. Many will not have been in touch with any clinics, and will not be on any maintenance or reducing programmes.

It is unusual to find self-help structures or support groups as drug users are not usually as well organised as, for example, gay men often are. However, there will usually be a *network of friends* or people with whom the drug user has relationships, often stormy, sometimes supportive and interdependent. These relationships are, of course, of continuing importance, whatever the stresses, when someone is increasingly ill or debilitated. Wherever the care is given, the needs of those who are close to the patient must also be borne in mind; although the needs of the patient must of course remain paramount, the carer may need some protection from time to time from their demands. In a hospice or hospital setting these stormy relationships may be difficult to contain in such a way as to minimise trauma and disruption to other patients. It is important, in planning services of care for this client group, to plan for an environment and policies which will accommodate potential problems such as those outlined above. Some may feel that services which are set up specifically for drug users by those with experience are more likely to be able to accommodate their needs. However, not all drug users would wish to be 'lumped together' when they need care, especially in the more advanced stages of the disease.

Homelessness is a specific issue which is faced by many drug users. The uncertainties inherent in their drug use and in homelessness renders risk reduction and the delivery of medical, nursing and social care particularly difficult (Lenkefeld et al., 1990, pp. 210 f).

Good nutrition and hygiene are often impossible to maintain, especially with increasing debility and illness. Patients are often lost to follow-up, and the conditions in which many drug users die may be very distressing. Many homeless people who are drug users with AIDS will also display the conditions common amongst the general homeless population in any city, such as trauma, infestations, behaviour problems, mental instability, peripheral vascular disease, and skin infections.

The needs of *women with children* in this situation are particularly poignant. Of the 273 paediatric AIDS cases reported to the New York City Department of Health in February 1988, approximately 73 per cent were known to have parents of whom one or both were known to be IDUs (Lenkefeld et al., 1990, p. 213). Women drug users may present late for care for many reasons; these may include a sense of guilt or the fear that the child or children will be taken into care if her own state becomes known. It is important where resources allow to plan special provisions which will, as far as possible, maintain the integrity of the family when one or more members of it are ill or dying (see also Chapter 12).

Clinical issues

Even in advanced HIV disease or AIDS, many drug users will continue to use drugs intravenously, sometimes regularly, often intermittently and on impulse in response to stress. Their case is therefore often complicated by unpredictable behaviour changes, and the constant need for negotiation about drugs, with the patient's or client's expressed need for opiates for pain relief or tranquillisers for anxiety and stress. The client's perception of need and that of the medical team may differ markedly. Medical and nursing personnel must guard against pre-judging the situation as 'yet another attempt to twist my arm for more opiates'. They must be vigilant to pick up early signs of unprescribed drug use, and must have a policy to deal consistently but compassionately with such situations. It may be a sign that pain or other symptoms, or fear, are not adequately being addressed. It is also important to bear in mind the possibility of drug interactions or overdosage. The patient or client who feels he or she is not being taken seriously, or is not being heard, may find it necessary to prove the existence of pain or the overwhelming nature of a stress, sometimes through a dramatic gesture.

To stabilise or to stop – that is often the question. Some centres will feel that a drug user must, at all costs, be encouraged to stop his drug use. Others, and increasingly those involved with HIV infected drug users, are convinced that it is more important to help the client to minimise harm and transmission of HIV, and to maintain stability as far as possible in those who are infected. The stress of stopping drug use may in itself be destructive to patients who have AIDS and who are already seriously debilitated. It may therefore be more important to work with the client to stabilise his drug use through, for example, a methadone maintenance programme, where methadone is used as a substitute for injected opiates. Injectable opiates or methadone may also be prescribed, with disposable needles and syringes. Other drugs, such as benzodiazepines, should then also be prescribed on a maintenance basis. Once the client is assured that there will be no reduction or stopping of his 'normal requirements', he is more likely to trust the practitioner, and to cooperate with other necessary medications. However, the prescriber should remember, even when trust seems to have been established, that the client is often habitually manipulative, may be obtaining prescriptions elsewhere, may be selling drugs to others and may still, from time to time, have the impulse to inject illicit drugs. It is important to negotiate or in some cases to state the boundaries of acceptable behaviour. Work towards establishing 'con-tracts' should include agreements about behaviour and reassurance about care and symptom control in those with advanced disease. Fear of pain, loss of independence and death may be at the root of some of the behaviour problems and should be discussed and explored when appropriate.

Much excellent work is being undertaken by agencies whose aims are harm reduction and prevention of HIV transmission, but these issues are not dealt with in this book. The reader is referred to the references and to the 'Further Reading' section for further information.

Symptom control in patients who are already 'loaded'

The *British National Formulary*, published by the British Medical Association with the Royal Pharmaceutical Society of Great Britain, in its issue of March 1993 makes the following statement on p. 180:

> Although caution is necessary, addicts (and ex-addicts) may be treated with analgesics in the same way as other people when there is a real clinical need. Doctors are reminded that (in Britain) they do not require a special licence to prescribe opioid analgesics for addicts for relief of pain due to organic disease or injury.

It is, indeed, important to remember that drug users ARE like other people in that they suffer the same range of symptoms and do experience pain in the same way that non-drug users do. However, because they are used to taking regular opioids or other drugs, they may require much larger doses of analgesics and anxiolytics to obtain the same effect. Patients on maintenance programmes are relatively easy to deal with when it comes to working out their requirements for relief of a new pain or problem. However, it may be more complex when dealing with patients who only use intermittently or who have not used drugs for some time, but the same basic principles apply.

Patients on methadone maintenance programmes

Patients will usually be taking methadone linctus daily or twice daily. Methadone is longer acting (having a longer plasma half-life) than morphine and there is a danger of accumulation if taken more frequently or in prolonged use. It can also be prescribed as tablets or as an injection for IV use.

Pain should be assessed and measured as in other patients, and analgesia should be prescribed in addition to the regular maintenance dose of methadone. In some countries or centres, additional metha-done, which is an excellent analgesic in itself, will be prescribed for opioid-responsive pain. In others, morphine elixir will be prescribed when appropriate. As in other patients, the effective dose is titrated in the same way as described in Chapter 6. The maintenance programme and the treatment of pain are thus seen as two separate issues. The risk of confusion is lessened by this approach. It should be remembered that patients will experience the side effects of morphine, such as nausea, while the doses are titrated upwards, and will often need an anti-emetic during this process. Remember, too, to prescribe a laxative to prevent or deal with constipation and explain its importance, though patients will usually be familiar with this problem. When a patient becomes unable to take oral medication, and if a syringe driver is required (see Chapter 6), the calculation of the diamorphine (or morphine) required over 24 hours should include the equivalent * of the oral methadone the patient has been taking. Similarly, when a patient has been taking benzodiaze-pines, remember to include their equivalent in calculating the total of midazolam required in the syringe driver to prevent a withdrawal reaction such as a seizure (see also p.86).

References

Antonucci, G., Girardi, E., Armignacco, O, et al. (1992). Tuberculosis in HIV-infected subjects in Italy with a multicentre study. AIDS 3(9) 1007–13.

British National Formulary (March 1993). British Medical Association and Royal Pharmaceutical Society of Great Britain.

Des Jarlais, D.C., Friedman, S.R., Choopanya, K. et al. (1992). International epidemiology of HIV and AIDS among injecting drug users. AIDS, 6 1053–68.

Greenberg, A.E., Thomas, P.A., Landesman, S.H., et al. (1992). The spectrum of HIV-1-related disease among outpatients in New York City. AIDS 6(9) 849–59.

Lenkefeld, C.G., Battjes, R.J., Amsel, Z. (Eds) (1990). AIDS and Intravenous Drug Use. Hemisphere Publishing Corporation.

Mientjes, G.H.C., Van Ameijden, E.X., Mulder, J.W. (1992). Prevalence of thrombocy-topenia in HIV-infected and non-infected drug users and homosexual men. British Journal of Haematology, 8293, 615–19.

Selwyn, P.A., Sckell, B.M., Alcabes, P. et al. (1992). High risk of active tuberculosis in HIV-infected drug users with cutaneous anergy. Journal of the American Medical Association, 268(4) 504–9.

Twycross, R. and Lack, S. (1990). Therapeutics in Terminal Cancer, second edition. Churchill Livingstone, Edinburgh.

* A single oral dose of 5 mg methadone is equivalent to morphine 7.5 mg (diamorphine 5 mg) and when given regularly is 3–4 times more potent and has a duration of action of 8–12 hours (Twycross and Lack, 1990).

11

Terminal care for women with HIV disease*

She had a diagnosis of chronic cryptosporidiosis with persistent diarrhoea, and also of pulmonary tuberculosis which was proving to be resistant to treatment. She had lost 10 kg in weight in the past few weeks and was suffering from chronic vaginal and oral candidiasis and her menstrual pattern had become irregular. She tended to focus on her gynaecological problems and she was depressed. She was anxious about her ten year old son's future and about who would take care of him as she had no family in the UK. Her husband had been killed in Africa and she had fled to the UK as a refugee with her son three years previously.

She had been struggling on at home refusing to be admitted because of Peter until she collapsed, dehydrated as a result of an acute exacerbation of diarrhoea and was admitted to hospital. Her son had been caring for her at home and called an ambulance. He was taken into care, to the same foster mother with whom he had spent a previous admission and with whom Sarah had maintained contact.

Having been rehydrated, stabilised and re-assessed at the acute hospital, Sarah was referred to Mildmay for terminal care where Peter continued to visit her daily. She was emaciated, depressed but in denial about her condition. She had not been able to discuss Peter's future in the event of her death – attempts by counsellors and social workers had met with denial or evasion of the problem. She was afraid to let any friends know the diagnosis, and she was afraid that Peter would be stigmatised at school should her status become known, although he was HIV negative.

When Sarah was found to have a perianal abscess causing her severe pain and distress, she was referred for surgery. Her

*Most of the material in this chapter has been reproduced by kind permission from *Women and HIV Disease*, published by Churchill Livingstone, 1993. Eds. M. Johnson & F. Johnstone.

own acute centre was unable to find a surgeon who was willing to deal with it, and she was therefore referred to another centre to which she was admitted for a few days. Unfortunately, she developed a rectovaginal fistula. Sadly, Peter was not allowed to visit as it was felt it would unsuitable for such a young child to see her in her condition post-operatively. Sarah became convinced that he had died and became acutely distressed and agitated. The psychiatrist who was called to see her did not understand her distress because of a language problem and diagnosed an acute psychosis, possibly relating to the general anaesthesia she had undergone.

When Sarah returned to Mildmay she was still acutely distressed, and wanted only to die. As soon as it became clear that she thought Peter was dead, arrangements were quickly made for Peter to visit. Peter had been very withdrawn and silent and he told the counsellor during his first visit that he had thought his mother had died since he could no longer visit her, and that everyone had been lying to him when they had reassured him.

Once Sarah and Peter were re-united, Sarah settled down. She continued to deteriorate, however, and it was felt that Peter should spend as much time as possible with her and he was allowed to stay with her on several occasions. Sarah began to be willing to explore issues relating to Peter's future with the nurses and the counsellor, and she also welcomed pastoral support from the chaplaincy team who arranged regular services of communion for her. Her physical symptoms of pain, nausea and diarrhoea were controlled and she died in peace and comfort, with her son by her side, and supported by the team. There had been some discussion about the distress to Peter of seeing other ill people on the ward, but Peter showed clearly that he coped well. He was happier helping to care for his mother than being separated from her. After Sarah's death, he returned to the foster mother who had supported him throughout.

Sarah's story illustrates a number of the issues surrounding terminal care for women with AIDS. These include some of the following:

- The clinical needs for palliation and/or acute treatment of distressing physical problems, some of which may be gynaecological in nature.
- Neuropsychiatric problems.

- The social isolation and fear with which many live with little of no support from family.
- The anxieties relating to child care and the future of orphans who may be left destitute in some societies.
- The need to provide support in the community for women who are themselves ill, and mothers in particular. This includes provision for flexible respite care and fostering arrangements, keeping separation to a minimum for the sake of both, and yet recognising that the mother will also need a break from the child from time to time.
- The needs of women who are usually 'the carers' needing care themselves. Who will care for them, when they are disabled, or ill or when they are dying?
- The need for ongoing financial support or for income generation. In many instances the woman will have been the sole breadwinner.
- Emotional, spiritual and pastoral needs.
- Confidentiality for herself and her child/children.
- The responsibilities of the woman as a carer for husband, elderly parents and children, without (in many countries) the power or right to make her own decisions and choices, even when it comes to matters of sexual intercourse, childbearing or the future of dependents.

Clinical problems

In most central African countries and in some areas of pattern I countries, for example in New York City, AIDS has become the leading cause of death for women aged 20–40 (Chin, 1990). Most will be dying with little or no access to medical help or even palliative care. Even in pattern I countries, such as the USA, and other Western areas where medical care is more readily available to all, women tend to delay in coming forward for medical care for themselves (*Triple Jeopardy* 1990). They are likely, therefore, to present with more advanced immunosuppression, and in a state of chronic ill health or as acute emergencies, unless they are fortunate enough to have been identified at an early stage and to have found medical and social support for themselves and their families.

Women with late stage HIV disease or AIDS are subject to a range of gynaecological problems which may cause anxiety, discomfort and pain, and exacerbate the ill health or weakness the patient is already experiencing as a result of HIV. Common gynaecological problems are, of course, common in this group of patients too, and it may not be possible to attribute their presence specifically to the HIV infection but more to immunosuppression and generally debility. These problems may include pelvic inflammatory disease, menstrual irregularities, genital warts and ulcers, chronic vaginal candidiasis and cervical dysplasia.

Candidiasis

Vaginal and oral or oesophageal candidiasis may cause severe debility and discomfort in someone who has advanced HIV disease. It may become increasingly difficult to control. Oral candidiasis will cause anorexia, loss of taste and in some cases soreness of oral mucosa with sensitivity to hot and cold liquids. This will cause loss of weight as the anorexia and loss of taste persist, thus increasing the debility. Oesophageal candidiasis may cause dysphagia and retrosternal discomfort with a burning sensation, not usually described as pain. Again, weight loss will become an increasing problem as nausea, vomiting, anorexia and dysphagia may be very troublesome.

Treatment of candidiasis, whether oral, oesophageal or vaginal, may be complicated by the need to treat bacterial infections with antibiotics. *Candida albicans* sometimes develops resistance to the usual drugs in patients with advanced disease, and even larger doses than normal may not then control the problems. Fluconazole is the treatment of choice in dosages which may range from 100 to 400 mg daily (Laine *et al.*, 1992). Ketaconazole 200 mg – 400 mg daily may also be used or in some cases itraconazole 200 mg daily, which may also be taken as a liquid. Very occasionally, amphotericin B or fluconazole may have to be given intravenously in someone with resistant oesophageal candida where symptoms of dysphagia and burning are causing distress; burning and itching due to vaginal candidiasis may also be distressing.

Nystatin suspension may contribute to the control of *oral candidiasis*, but larger doses than those normally recommended are required in patients with severe immunosuppression (Meunier-Carpentier, 1984). A dose of 3–5 ml should be given every 2–4 hours, and held in the mouth for as long as possible before swallowing. Unfortunately some patients may develop diarrohea as a side effect or may find the taste unpleasant. Nystatin or amphotericin pastilles may then be sucked instead. Miconazole tablets 250 mg may also be sucked, and miconazole oral gel (Daktarin R), which is sugarless, may be more acceptable to some patients. In very resistant cases, clotrimazole (Canestan) vaginal tablets, (100, 200 or 500 mg) taken orally and sucked once or twice daily, may be effective in clearing plaques of oral candidiasis within 2–3 days; some patients find the taste and foaming of the tablets unpleasant in the mouth, but may be pleasantly surprised to find quick relief.

Vaginal candidiasis may be similarly distressing and difficult to treat in severely immunosuppressed women. Systemic treatment with fluconazole or other drugs mentioned above will be necessary, with the application of clotrimazole cream to the vulva and clotrimazole vaginal tablets inserted as high as possible in the vagina. Tablets of 500 mg will be more effective than the lower dosages in controlling symptoms quickly.

Recurrences of infection are almost inevitable, and most patients will require *prophylactic* or *maintenance* treatment with, for example, fluconazole. In advanced disease, higher doses will be required to maintain control. Perianal candida infections and other skin sites, such as groin, umbilicus or under the breasts, may also require regular attention with clotrimazole or miconazole cream.

In the *terminal care* situation the patient may be unable to take oral medication. Here the administration of nystatin suspension or miconazole oral gel (with good mouth care) is even more important in order to maintain comfort. Vulvitis and vaginitis should not be forgotten as a possible cause of restlessness in a dying patient or of dysuria and frequency, and treated appropriately. Natural yoghurt may be soothing when applied to the vulva, and, taken orally, may help to control oral or oesophageal candidiasis.

Cervical dysplasia

Cervical abnormalities are common in women infected with HIV (Norman *et al.*, 1990) and recent studies have shown that there is a high risk of human papillomavirus (HPV) infection and cervical intraepithelial lesions among women with advanced HIV-related disease (Vermund *et al.*, 1991). Another study suggests that the increased risk for the development of neoplasia of the uterine cervix in women with HIV infection is related to the degree of immunosuppression (Schafer *et al.*, 1991). Immunosuppression may stimulate or exacerbate the development of HPV-related condylomata acuminata and lead to an increased incidence of cervical carcinoma. It appears that more advanced HIV infection is associated with a greater risk of these abnormalities (Esplin and Levine, 1991).

Genital herpes simplex infections

Genital herpes infections become progressively more common as the CD4+ lymphocyte count falls. There is often a high rate of previous sexually transmitted diseases (Norman *et al.*, 1990). The association between genital ulcerative disease and HIV infection is well established (Cameron and Padian, 1990; Plourde *et al.*, 1992).

Herpes ulceration may cause severe stinging and burning of the vulva or vagina, with dysuria. In patients with advanced disease, the lesions may be difficult to treat effectively. Acyclovir given orally in doses of 400 mg five times daily, with the local application of acyclovir cream where possible, will promote healing and relief within a week to ten days when resistance has not developed. When the ulceration persists despite treatment, distress and agitation may become difficult to deal with, and patients may require analgesia in the form of morphine with an anxiolytic or sedative. (See further under 'Symptom control issues', p. 80f.). Local anaesthetic gels may give relief for a while, but prolonged regular applications may cause local sensitivity reactions. Some patients will find relief from soaking in a mildly saline bath. Patients who are too weak even for this require careful and meticulous attention to hygiene by the nursing staff (see also p. 66).

In patients who have well advanced HIV disease with emaciation, weakness and immobility, pressure areas may break down and become infected with herpes, causing extensive ulceration of sacral or perianal areas or around the vulva. Severe distress and pain is the result and must be managed with good wound care, treatment of infection where possible, and regular and adequate analgesia with morphine and/or nonsteroidal anti-inflammatory medications. A short-acting but effective analgesic may be given prior to wound dressings, such as dextromoramide 5–10 mg orally or by injection. Alternatively, if the patient is on a syringe driver with diamorphine, a boost may be given just before the procedure. Entonox (50 per cent mixture of nitrous oxide and oxygen) may be helpful in some patients during painful procedures. (See also under 'Symptom control issues', p. 77).

Pelvic inflammatory disease

This is very common in women who are at risk of sexually transmitted diseases. It may result in severe lower abdominal pain, and cause confusion in the differential diagnosis of abdominal emergencies. In advanced AIDS chronic problems may cause increasing debility and discomfort and should be managed so as to promote comfort and pain relief as far as possible. Constipation may also cause lower abdominal pain; this is particularly likely in someone on regular opioid analgesia, and should be prevented with regular stool softeners, such as lactulose.

Tuberculosis

In countries where tuberculosis is widespread there is a marked association between HIV and tuberculosis, with a resurgence of multiple drug resistant tuberculosis associated with problems in some Western countries, e.g. the USA (Fischl et al., 1992). It is expected that pelvic tuberculosis will also increase (Norman et al., 1990), as indeed will other pelvic inflammatory diseases. In end-stage disease, treatment with dexamethasone may reduce the pain or discomfort associated with pelvic and abdominal tuberculosis (see also p. 61ff.).

Pregnancy

Although the evidence does not suggest a significant effect on the outcome of pregnancy in HIV seropositive women or that pregnancy accelerates the disease progression (Newell *et al.*, 1990), it has been shown that HIV seropositive women with low CD4 counts (below 300 cells/cu.mm are markedly at risk of serious infections during pregnancy (Minkoff *et al.*, 1990) (see further in *Women and HIV Disease* 1993; see also Chapter 12).

Intravenous drug users

As many HIV infected women in the West are intravenous drug users, many of the problems they face are related to their drug use. These may be social and medical. Patients with the weakness and debility associated with well advanced AIDS or HIV disease often appear to become less dependent on the drugs as they become more dependent on nursing care. However, in treating the patient's pain it is important to bear in mind the past history and pattern of drug use and to adjust the dosages appropriately. For example, patients who have already been on opiates, albeit not prescribed, may need larger than the usual dosages to deal effectively with pain. The same applies to benzodiazepines such as diazepam or temazepam for anxiolysis or night sedation. In the terminal care situation it is more important to treat pain and other symptoms effectively than to be concerned to treat or prevent addiction. Maintenance doses of methadone will enable the patient to remain stable, while any pain problems should be treated separately and appropriate and adequate analgesia or adjuvant treatment given (see Chapter 10).

Median survival times

In overall terms, median survival times in women who are not receiving zidovudine or didanosine are shorter than in men after diagnosis of AIDS. In recent years overall survival times for all patients have improved (Lemp *et al.*, 1992). As women tend to present later for diagnosis and treatment, and may have less easy access to care in some countries, it may be that immunosuppression through HIV infection has progressed further at the point of presentation in these women (*Triple Jeopardy*, 1990).

This may mean that some women will have a shorter time period in which to come to terms with their own losses and fears about the physical progress of the disease. The same applies to dealing with the many social issues and decisions which have to be faced (see section on 'Social needs'), in particular to planning for the future of any children.

Neuropsychiatric problems

A variety of neuropsychiatric problems occur in advanced AIDS which range from acute anxiety to frank psychoses, extreme paranoia and dementia. Depression and anxiety are very common and may be masked by organic disease processes, including HIV encephalopathy. What role a developing HIV encephalopathy plays in the development of post-morbid psychiatric syndromes is not clear. One study in Zaire showed that 41 per cent of HIV seropositive patients showed evidence of neuropsychiatric abnormalities (Perriens et al., 1992). One post-mortem study showed that nearly 90 per cent of patients reviewed had cerebral abnormalities (Lantos et al., 1989). An unpublished analysis of 100 patients admitted consecutively to a hospice unit (Mildmay Mission Hospital) revealed that 22 per cent had a significant psychiatric problem other than mild anxiety or depression. The same range of neurological problems occur in women as in men.

Women with neuropsychiatric problems who also have children present special problems. It is distressing for the child to watch its mother behaving in bizarre and uncharacteristic ways, which may also be very frightening. Counsellors and social workers seeking to help the mother to deal with issues relating to her own impending death and her child's future may have difficulties with enabling her to reach meaningful resolutions. Great sensitivity, patience and an ability to work with children and other family members are essential.

Patients with advance AIDS appear to be more sensitive than usual to psychotropic drugs and smaller doses than those normally recommended for the treatment of psychiatric problems may be required to avoid serious sedation and extrapyramidal side effects. However, in seriously disturbed or psychotic patients it may be necessary to use high doses to achieve control. In a terminally ill patient methotrimeprazine or midazolam may be used in the syringe driver to control severe agitation and restlessness (Black, 1992) (see also Chapter 6).

Social needs and problems

Someone to care for her

Women are usually the providers of care for husbands, children and elderly parents. The woman who has a partner willing to care for her when she herself is ill, disabled or dying is indeed fortunate. Sadly there are many women who are deserted by their partner when they are no longer able to fulfil their usual role or when the diagnosis becomes known. In cultures where the extended family system is strong, such as in Scotland or Uganda, the task of caring for the ill woman will usually fall to her mother. In some cultures the woman will be expected to move back into her parental home with her children if they are small. Thus, the grandmother will often become the surrogate mother for the children. Grandmothers are the main carers in many communities in Africa where large numbers of women of childbearing age are dying as a result of AIDS. This places a huge burden on elderly women who may themselves be suffering from the problems of increasing age. In the West, with many women living far from their parents, often being themselves single parents, there may be no-one to care for the ill or dying woman who will end up in hospital unless community services can be set up to provide care in the home.

Delays in treatment

The responsibility for a child or children, and the resistance the woman may have to the child being taken into care may cause her to delay in seeking help. The situation may then become an emergency and result in admission to hospital with the children taken into care amidst great trauma. Other reasons for delay may be guilt about a lifestyle such as drug misuse, guilt about 'being the cause' of the child's HIV status, guilt about 'not being able to cope' and a resultant feeling that she does not deserve help. In one study in New York, women were found to be already very ill when they first presented for medical treatment. On average, women suffered nearly 60 weeks of ill health before seeking medical care, compared with just 24 in men (*Triple Jeopardy*, 1990).

Confidentiality

Other anxieties often relate to issues of confidentiality. Once her HIV status is known to social services, home help services or her GP, to whom else will the knowledge be 'leaked'? What will be the result for her child? Will he or she be ostracised, stigmatised, and be thrown out of school or creche? What about the neighbours?

One mother with AIDS attended a day centre to which she was given a lift in a car which had the name of an institution well known for its AIDS care on the side. She would also be taken back and dropped off outside her home in a block of flats. She would then go to the nearby school to bring her daughter home from school. One day, as they approached their block, a bucket of water was thrown over them from an upstairs flat. Subsequent events convinced her that neighbours had observed the name on the car and put two and two together. She requested that the name be removed from the car to prevent similar problems happening to other people.

The fear of confidentiality being broken may have a profound effect on the woman's attitudes to her own need for medical help. Here, fear of the reactions she or her child may provoke if the diagnosis becomes known may keep her isolated and lacking in the support and help that could be available to her.

The need for respite and support in the community

A woman who is herself debilitated, disabled or ill whilst still caring for a small child will suffer extreme fatigue and exhaustion at times, particularly as her condition advances. It is important to plan for support for her in the community or for flexible respite admissions with arrangements for the child to remain with the mother should she wish for this. Provisions should then be made for the child to be cared for by, for example, nursery nurses during the day and, perhaps also at night, to give the mother adequate periods of rest.

Other forms of support could include creche facilities for children under five so that the woman can have several 'free' periods during the week. A flexible approach to this may also be helpful so that, if she feels particularly unwell one day, the child may be taken to the creche or to a foster mother. This may enable her to cope in the community for as long as possible, even when suffering chronic ill health.

Fostering and adoption

In Scotland an innovative approach to fostering has been developed to support mothers who have advanced AIDS. Prospective foster parents are trained in issues relating to HIV/AIDS and may be introduced to a mother soon after her first admission with an AIDS-related condition (Brettle, 1990). The foster mother is then allocated to that family 'on standby'. During subsequent admissions of the mother to hospital the child is then cared for by the same foster mother so that both mother and child become secure in the knowledge of the arrangement. As the mother's condition advances, discussions may then begin about arrangements for the child when she dies.

Similarly, prospective adoptive parents may also be given some training in regard to HIV/AIDS. For some mothers it is important to have an opportunity to meet the people who may adopt her child after her death. Others will not be able to cope with this, and in some cultures it is only felt appropriate for the child to go to a member of the extended family. For example, in Zimbabwe, some families will be unwilling to introduce into the 'family line' a child from an unrelated family as he or she may bring misfortune or 'a curse' upon the adoptive family. It is felt the child may be blamed for any subsequent problems which could arise. Thus, in this situation, some may prefer orphans to go into an orphanage. In Uganda, however, it is felt that the community should take responsibility for its orphans. Great sensitivity is needed in broaching the subject with an ill or dying woman, together with some understanding of her cultural background.

Emotional and spiritual care

Children, illness and death

Women who have lost a considerable amount of weight, who are disfigured, who have developed signs of HIV encephalopathy or who have psychiatric problems may cause a great deal of distress to their partner or children as their condition deteriorates. Some women will not wish their child to see them in this condition – they will wish the child to 'remember me as I was'. The partner and adult family members, will make their own decisions about how much time they spend with the dying woman, and whether or not they wish to be with her at the moment of death, bearing in mind her need for supportive company.

However, a small child is in a different situation. Some mothers may make it clear that they do not wish the child to see them; others, like Sarah, will be very distressed by separation. Some children, like Peter, will be happier to be involved, and will cope well. Great sensitivity is needed in supporting both the dying woman and the family through this time. Nursing, medical, social work, counselling and pastoral personnel will all be involved, and will need to work together to develop a common approach in each individual case.

Counselling

Counselling will, in most instances, focus around the issues already discussed. The woman who faces all the losses inherent in being someone with advanced AIDS will require understanding support which enables her, where possible, to make meaningful decisions. In many cultures, particularly in developing countries, women are not empowered to make decisions for themselves about any major issues, including their children's future. They may therefore be unused to, or afraid of, broaching or discussing difficult emotional issues. In some Kenyan circles, for example, it is considered unacceptable to discuss someone's impending death as this, in itself, is seen as hastening or causing the death. Therefore, a wife who has the courage or temerity to raise the subject of her own or her husband's possible death with a view to making decisions about the children's future support may be accused of causing the death. She may even be thrown out of the home and disinherited by the rest of the family. A counsellor faced with such a cultural background will have to be prepared to approach the whole subject in a roundabout, indirect way, and may need to be very patient, accepting the cultural inability of the ill woman to deal with the issue.

The question of wills may also cause similar problems. In the West, counsellors dealing with a person in the terminal phase of her illness would naturally raise the issue and provide supportive help to someone seeking to complete 'unfinished business', such as the writing of a will. A woman would be encouraged to do this in the same way that a man would be.

However, in many cultures it would be seen as inappropriate for a woman to do so, and in some a will written by a woman would not be considered legally binding in any case. She may not be able to own anything in her own name, and therefore will have nothing to leave. These issues are now being addressed in many developing countries where the writing of any wills has not been common. Tribal law will have dictated what happens to property or money after someone's death. For example, in Ugandan common law, the husband's brothers inherit any property he leaves. In parts of Uganda women lawyers are encouraging women to take control of their own situations and seek legal advice about how to write a legally valid will. Women with AIDS who have been able to set up income generating projects are opening accounts in the names of their children to ensure some continuing financial support for them. Men are also being encouraged to plan ahead and to write wills which will provide ongoing support for their spouse and children. However, these are still new ideas for some communities and cannot be imposed.

Counsellors may therefore have to work with women to whom the whole idea of writing a will, and making decisions relating to their own death, may be very unfamiliar, even shocking. Emotionally, a woman may not be able to handle the issue and may therefore avoid or deny the need to do so.

Pastoral care

A woman's religious background may be or become very important at this time. Even someone with little or no religious affiliation will begin to ask questions which have spiritual significance, and some will discover a faith for the first time. It is vitally important that spiritual issues and questions relating to the meaning of life, suffering and death be taken seriously. Pastoral care should be available through a chaplaincy team or contact be made with religious leaders from her own background. Religious rites and practices may take on a meaning and an importance they have not had until the woman became ill, particularly during the terminal phase.

The family or the woman herself may express strong wishes with regard to the funeral; a chaplain should be available to discuss these wishes, and to enable them to be fulfilled as far as possible.

It is also important to bear in mind that spiritual conflict or pain may have a profound effect on symptoms and on the response to symptom control measures. A person who feels that her illness or pain is a punishment for something in the past is in great need of spiritual help. She may feel she should bear the pain stoically as a punishment or that she does not deserve to be given any relief or help. She needs to feel forgiven by God, by the people she feels she has wronged, and also by herself. A woman who has an HIV-positive child may feel very guilty about having infected her child or about leaving her family orphaned.

Anger or anxiety may also affect the response to proffered help, to medication and to the perception of symptoms. The anger may be directed at God or at the religious community from which the person comes; anxiety may be about what will/may happen after death. The reality and depth of these feelings must not be negated or ignored. Good teamwork between doctors, nurses and spiritual careers may result in resolution of fears and relief of problems or symptoms, leading to a death marked by peace instead of conflict.

Conclusion

In addition to the physical problems that anyone with AIDS faces, a woman may have gynaecological problems requiring urgent diagnosis and treatment. However, she will also be facing a number of issues that are of special concern to her – as a childbearer, a mother, a wife and a daughter. As the disease process advances and death approaches, these issues become more acute. The question arises of who will care for her, the one who is usually the carer, when she is too weak to cope or when acute illness or terminal problems overtake her. And who will care for those whom she usually supports – her children, her elderly parents, her husband or partner, who may also be ill?

The memories with which the woman's family, partner and children are left will be profoundly coloured by the attitudes of the whole team at this crucial time. The medical and nursing problems, the distress or conflict in which she may die if appropriate, skilled support is not available will remain with them for ever. In such a case, anger, bitterness or fear may be the legacy that a poorly managed death will leave with the survivors. On the other hand, when symptoms are well controlled, when anxiety or fear is alleviated, when appropriate plans are made with the woman, and when spiritual comfort and reassurance are available, the patient will be more likely to die with dignity and in peace. The memories then, even in the midst of grief, can bring comfort and strength for the future.

References

Back, I.N. (1992). Terminal restlessness in patients with advanced malignant disease. *Palliative Medicine*, **6** 293–8.

Brettle, R. (1990). Personal communication.

Cameron, W.D. and Padian, N.S. (1990). Sexual transmission of HIV and the epidemiology of other sexually transmitted diseases. *AIDS*, **4** (Suppl 1) S99–S103.

Chin, J. (1990). Current and future dimensions of the HIV/AIDS pandemic in women and children. *Lancet*, **336** 221–4.

Esplin, J.A. and Levine, A.M. (1991). HIV related neoplastic disease: 1991. *AIDS*, **5** (Suppl 2) S203–S210.

Fischl, M.A., Uttamchandani, R.B., Daikos, G.L. *et al.* (1992). An outbreak of tuberculosis caused by multiple drug resistant tubercle bacilli among patients with HIV infection. *Annals of Internal Medicine* **117(3)** 177–83.

Johnson, I. (1992). Drugs used in combination in the syringe driver – a survey of hospice practice. *Palliative Medicine*, **6** 125–30.

Laine, W., Dretler, R.H., Conteas, C.N. *et al.* (1992). Fluconazole compared with ketoconazole for the treatment of candida oesophagitis in AIDS – a randomised trial. *Annals of Internal Medicine*, **117(8)** 655–60.

Lantos, P.L., McLaughlin, J.E., Scholtz, C.L. *et al.* (1989). Neuropathology of the brain in HIV infection. *Lancet*, **1 (8633)**, 309.

Lemp, G.F., Hirozawa, A.M., Cohen, J.B. *et al.* (1992). Survival for women and men with AIDS. *Journal of Infectious Diseases*, **166(1)** 74–9.

Meunier-Carpentier, F. (1984). Chemoprophylaxis of fungal infection. *American Journal of Medicine*, **76**, 652–6.

Minkoff, H.L., Willoughby, A., Mendez, H. (1990). Serious infections during pregnancy among women with advanced HIV infection. *American Journal of Obstetrics and Gynecology*, **162(1)**, 30–4.

Moss, V.A. (1990). Palliative care in advanced HIV disease: presentation, problems and palliation. *AIDS*, **4** (Suppl 1) S235–S242.

Mulvenna, P. and Moss, V.A. (1990). AIDS related diarrhoea: a rational approach to symptomatic treatment. *Palliative medicine*, **6** 261. (Corresp.)

Newell, M.L., Peckham, C., Lepage, P. (1990). HIV infection in pregnancy: implications for women and children. *AIDS*, **4** (Suppl (1)) S111–S17.

Norman, S., Studd, J., Johnson, M. (1990). HIV infection in women. *British Medical Journal*, **301** 1231–2.

O'Neill, W. (1992). AIDS related diarrhoea: a rational approach to symptomatic treatment. *Palliative Medicine*, **6** 61–4.

Perriens, J.H., Mussa, M., Luabeya, M.K. *et al.* (1992). Neurological complications of HIV seropositive internal medicine patients in Kinshasa, Zaire. *Journal of AIDS*, **5(4)** 333–40.

Plourde, P.J., Plummer, F.A., Pepian, J. (1992). HIV-1 infection in women attending a sexually transmitted diseases clinic in Kenya. *Journal of Infectious Diseases*, **166(1)** 86–92.

Schafer, A., Friedmann, W., Mielke, M. (1991). The increased frequency of neoplasia in women infected with the HIV is related to the degree of immunosuppression. *American Journal of Obstetrics and Gynaecology*, **164(2)** 593–9.

Swerdlow, M. and Ventafridda, V. (Eds) (1987). *Cancer Pain*. MTP Press, Lancaster, UK.

Triple Jeopardy: Women and AIDS. (1990). The Panos Institute, London.

Vermund, S.H., Kelly, K.F., Klein, R.S. (1991). High risk of human papillomavirus infection and cervical squamous intraepithelial lesions among women with symptomatic HIV infection. *American Journal of Obstetrics and Gynecology*, **165(2)** 392–400.

Von Roenn, J.H. (1988). Megestrol acetate for treatment of cachexia associated with human immunodeficiency virus infection. *Annals of Internal Medicine*, **109** 840–1.

12

Care for families with HIV and AIDS

Care of mothers with AIDS

It remains a deeply felt need for some women to have children in spite of a diagnosis of AIDS. The estimate of transmission risk from mother to child varies from 13 per cent in the European Collaborative Study (1988–1991) to 39 per cent in African studies. For some, the possibility (61–87 per cent) (Hira *et al.* 1989) that the child will NOT be infected gives them sufficient hope to embark on pregnancy; many have no choice.

During pregnancy careful medical supervision, where possible, will be needed with supportive counselling to enable the mother to cope with the problems and uncertainties. Drug treatment for infections will be limited by the risks to the baby but against this will have to be weighed the mother's need for treatment.

When the baby is born the mother is confronted with the dilemma of whether to breastfeed or not. The following are the guidelines issued by the WHO and UNICEF in May 1992:

> Breastfeeding should be recommended to HIV infected areas where infectious diseases and malnutrition are the main causes of infant deaths. Where the main cause of infant deaths are not infectious diseases, a safe substitute for breast milk should be used.

In the West it is now possible to test the child within the first three months for infection, thus eliminating uncertainty. However, in most developing countries this is not possible and the first indication of infection will be that the child becomes symptomatic of HIV disease.

Many mothers with AIDS do not have a partner living with them so problems often arise when they are unwell:

- The lethargy and fatigue associated with HIV disease may affect them to such an extent that, at times, they do not have the energy to look after themselves, let alone care for a baby or small child.

- When the mother needs to be admitted to hospital for treatment, care for the child has to be organised. An emergency admission further compounds the problem.
- Patients who are immigrants or refugees often have no family or close friends who can help them in an emergency.
- The option of respite care will often not be acceptable if it means that the mother will be separated from her child. To be separated from a small child is difficult at any time but if it is known that your time together is limited it becomes even more distressing (see also Chapter 11).

Responses

In London some of the designated AIDS units are planning to provide for the needs of mothers with children by providing facilities that enable the child to stay with its mother when she is admitted to hospital.

Mothers who on occasions need help with caring for their children will benefit from day nursery places but need transport to be provided. In some areas child minders and foster parents are being trained to respond to these urgent needs. Some mothers would like help in the home to look after the child, whilst others feel that this is an invasion of their privacy.

Mildmay is now offering respite, rehabilitative and terminal care for families (when one or more family members have AIDS) in a purpose built family care centre. This comprises units for 12 families where facilities provide for the palliative care for adults and children and care for other affected family members. The mother can be as involved as she wishes, or is able, to be in the care of her child. The needs of infected and affected children are catered for with 24-hour care by qualified child care staff. The aim of this model of care is to enable families to stay together and, by providing respite admission, to support community care.

Karen is three years old. She has come into hospital for her three-weekly infusion of gamma globulin. In the cot next to her is two year old Emma. They and their parents know each other well as they have been coming in like this every three weeks since each was nine months old.

Karen and Emma are both quite small for their age with big hollow eyes, thin hair and dry skin. Karen accepts the hospital routine quite passively including the infusion needle in her arm. The infusion over, Karen is enjoying a bowl of strawberry ice cream while the paediatrician is talking to her mother. The doctor is explaining that she is going to give Karen zidovudine. Her T helper cell count is less than 300/cu. mm and the doctor is concerned that she will deteriorate very quickly. Karen's mother wonders whether she should be having zidovudine as well; she also has AIDS. She is feeling very tired and is very worried about what will happen to Karen if she is ill and cannot look after her, or if she dies before Karen does.

Children with AIDS

In the United Kingdom the number of children who have AIDS is still relatively small. Most of these children will be cared for, and ultimately will die in hospital. A few may die at home cared for by the parent(s) with back-up from the primary care team and/or specialist home care teams.

The common modes of transmission are

- from a mother who is HIV antibody positive
- through receiving contaminated blood and blood products
- through breast milk.

Children with AIDS commonly suffer from the following:

- *Pneumocystis carinii* pneumonia or lymphoid interstitial pneumonitis which cause dyspnoea and pyrexia.
- Candidiasis which may be recurrent and severe and cause difficulty with eating, as may herpes sores in and around the mouth.
- Intractable diarrhoea and severe weight loss.
- Recurrent opportunistic and bacterial infections.
- CNS involvement and encephalopathy may be evident in retarded development, spasticity, weakness and fits. (These children often need long term care).
- Failure to thrive.

Input to care for these children will be as for any child with a life threatening illness – an appropriate response to the individual needs of the child and his or her family. It is essential that the carers have a knowledge and understanding of paediatric AIDS, symptom control and palliative care. As all of the babies and children will have a mother with HIV disease, issues relating to fostering and adoption should be explored and options identified.

At the present time it is both possible and appropriate for children with AIDS to be cared for either in hospital or at home in the UK. There are, however, several factors that need to be considered if health care professionals are to continue to be able to respond effectively to the needs of these children and their families, as numbers grow:

- The longer term needs of children who are chronically sick.
- The fact that many mothers do not want to care for their children 'at home'.
- 'Home' may be a squat or bed and breakfast accommodation.
- Some mothers will be 'chaotic' drug users and be unable to care for a sick child.
- Chronically ill mothers with well or sick children will need help and respite.

The experience of colleagues in New York caring for large numbers of children with AIDS indicates that it is necessary to plan to provide longer term care for children. Terminal care facilities for children, as a back-up to community care, may also be needed. Planners of services within the statutory and voluntary sector need to talk to mothers who are HIV antibody positive, and carers already involved to identify what will be required and any likely gaps in service provision (see further in: *Children with HIV/AIDS* 1992. R. Claxton).

Children affected by AIDS

The needs of children affected by AIDS, but not infected, must not be overlooked.

- The child whose father has AIDS
- The child whose mother has AIDS
- The child whose sister/brother has AIDS.

Counselling teams in hospices are receiving increasing numbers of referrals of these children. The children need help to cope with the stigma and prejudice surrounding the diagnosis as well as issues related to loss, death and dying. Children may have become part of the conspiracy of silence surrounding the diagnosis of their family member, sworn to secrecy and unable to cope with the feelings of fear, guilt and shame.

If their brother or sister is sick and needing a lot of care and attention they may feel rejected and unloved and this may result in jealousy and attention-seeking behaviour. They need to be involved in the caring wherever possible, as this will enable them to feel valued and needed.

Some mothers have expressed the desire that their children should not see them when they are dying. They want to be remembered looking well. However, our experience is that when that situation arises premature goodbyes are not easy or often possible for the mother or the child.

Some older children have to cope with the realisation that not only does their father have AIDS but that he has been involved in homosexual or other relationships. If this happens during puberty they find it much more difficult to deal with. All too often the assumption is made that it is better not to involve children in painful or difficult situations. 'What they don't know, they won't worry about.' Our experience is that most children have a great capacity for understanding if issues are explained and opportunities given for questions and discussion. With small children play and art therapy may help them to explore and express their feelings.

Children are often in need of an advocate when a parent is dying or following the death of a parent. At this time the focus is inevitably on the patient and his or her needs and consideration of what is best for the child may be secondary.

It should also be remembered that families and children infected and affected by AIDS are not immune from the other problems that families may experience, e.g. sexual, physical and emotional abuse. Children may frequently be subjected to verbal abuse from parents who at times are overwhelmed with problems and find difficulty in coping.

This inconsistency may cause the child to be confused and fearful of 'outbursts', perhaps leading to constant anxiety, sleeping or behaviour problems or to withdrawal.

Grandparents

The care of most children who are orphaned in the UK at present is taken on by their grandparents. This is particularly true of patients who come from a drug using background and also from Africa. Grandparents are rising to the challenge, wanting to keep the child within the family circle. They also need special support, perhaps financially as well as emotionally and practically.

Adoption

When seeking adoptive parents outside the family the wishes of the parent and the needs of the children must be considered by people with expertise in this area.

When placing children there may be cultural and tribal issues that will affect the choice of adoptive parents. In our experience there is still a limited amount of expertise available in the HIV/child-care field, although more agencies are aware of the issues.

Other family members

When the family consists of a father, mother and other children the needs of the father and siblings must not be overlooked. Needs will vary depending on who the patient is and whether more than one family member has AIDS.

If mother is ill father will need support in caring for the children, maintaining the home and keeping the family together. He may have to give up work to do this which will probably have financial implications. If a child is ill then, as stated earlier, it is important not to make the other brothers and sisters feel left out and neglected. They also need to feel loved and supported in their sadness.

Terry was twelve years old when his older brother was admitted to the Mildmay for terminal care. Staff noticed that Terry often appeared distracted and a little anxious whilst visiting his brother. When asked if anything was worrying him Terry said there were a few 'silly things', as he put it, he would like to know about but didn't want to bother his parents.

One of the hospice counsellors came to see Terry. She found him eager to talk, asking lots of questions particularly about the process of death. 'How would we know when his brother was dying?' 'Was it possible for someone to be buried before they were actually dead?' 'How do you check that someone has died?' 'What happens to the body?' These were the so-called 'silly things' Terry was worried about. Counselling involved reassurance about practical details and time to explore his feeling about his brother's illness and impending death. Terry knew his brother had AIDS and was gay (that had never been a secret in their family), but there was a sense of isolation from his peers brought about by keeping the secret from his school friends. He had told them that his brother had cancer and often found it difficult to respond to their enquiries about his health.

It soon became clear that Terry's brother was a significant figure in his life, someone he admired and respected who would be sorely missed. The counsellor suggested that Terry might like to make a book about his brother and himself. Through this book many memories were shared, photographs and pictures were collected with the whole family contributing. Terry's brother contributed to the book only days before he died.

Terry continued to see the counsellor following his brother's death, and through continued work on his book he felt able to ask specific questions about HIV and AIDS, especially around transmission. He had taken to wearing some of his brother's clothes and thought that this might put him at risk from infection. He wanted more information about HIV and AIDS to help try to make sense of his brother's death. Through sensitive listening and support Terry was given time to explore issues at his own pace, and at his level of understanding. As with most children, his fantasy was often far worse than the reality.

Maintaining the family affected by AIDS as a unit is not always easy. The unpredictability of the disease and the need for urgent action places the family and statutory carers under immense pressure. However, we are learning how to cope with the problems and are seeking satisfactory outcomes where families, statutory and voluntary carers are working well together.

References

Claxton, R., and Harrison, A. (1990) *Caring for Children with HIV and AIDS*. Edward Arnold, London.

European Collaborative Study (1988). Mother and child transmission of HIV infection. *Lancet*, **ii**, 1039–42.

European Collaborative Study (1991). Children born to women with HIV infection: natural history and risk of transmission. *Lancet*, **337**, 253–60.

Hira, S.K., Kamanga, J., Bhat, G.J. *et al.* (1989). Perinatal transmission of HIV 1 in Zambia. *British Medical Journal*, **299**, 1250–2.

13

Care where resources are limited

'In order to have a real impact, preventative programmes must go hand in hand with care.'

Amina Ali, Chief Nurse, Tanzania, 1991

Introduction

In countries where resources are limited it is easy to understand the priority that is usually given to programmes of prevention and education, or counselling which is aimed at achieving sexual behaviour change in individuals or communities. However, even in the case of preventive messages, the greatest impact is often made when practical care and compassion are linked with education and demonstrated by example – 'your actions speak louder than your words'.

Very limited resources are often allocated to health; available resources are frequently diverted or given to other priorities, such as defence. Operation Desert Storm in the Middle East conflict cost $49 billion; in 1993 the WHO estimated that an effective prevention package for the world would cost $2.5 billion, barely one twentieth of the cost of the conflict, or the equivalent of 'one can of Coke for every person in the world' (Merson, 1993).

When health is prioritised, prevention of HIV is given a higher priority than care. However, the considerable numbers of people living with HIV and AIDS, if given support and care, still have much to contribute to society although they are often made to feel that they have been written off.

The truth is, people with AIDS or HIV are in the main young and productive, and are usually parents with small children who need them for as long as possible. Any efforts and resources that can be made available to care for those who are intermittently ill or to support those who are caring for someone who is chronically ill or dying will benefit present communities and future generations.

Existing health care problems

With health care spending at such a low level it is hardly surprising that in some parts of the world resources are inadequate to meet the existing health care needs of the populations. If the provision of *hospital care*, which is always expensive, is limited by inadequate finance this will affect the quality of the care provided in a number of ways including:

- poor maintenance of buildings/wards/equipment
- inadequate staffing levels in wards/departments
- drugs not available or inadequate supplies
- laboratory equipment for investigating patients not available
- limited training opportunities for staff
- limited availability of gloves, syringes, needles and other disposables.

The demand for services in some areas far exceeds the ability to respond, causing overcrowding in wards and clinics and a feeling of impotence for staff who have no treatment to offer. When care is being provided *in the community* there are additional problems that have to be faced:

- Access to services, such as clinics or hospitals may be difficult for sick patients
- Limited transport is available and access for visiting teams to some areas is impossible by car
- Once trained, the majority of nurses and other health care professionals demonstrate a preference for working in towns and cities. This causes staff shortage in clinics and teams working in rural areas.

Even where there are drugs and treatments available most patients are unable to afford to purchase them over a protracted period of time. As we know, many of the problems experienced in developing countries are the result of civil war, intertribal conflict and corruption. These are often set against a backdrop of poverty and famine. All over the world, fear, fuelled by ignorance and myths relating to HIV, inhibits progress in the provision of care to people with AIDS. Some health care professionals and carers who still fear transmission from mosquitoes and bugs, or by contact, are certainly not willing to touch or care for people with AIDS. In addition, the training programmes essential to dispel the myths and fears are not always available, even for health care professionals. Surprisingly, despite all this, excellent models of care for people with AIDS are being developed, often by non-government and self-help organisations. Even in most government institutions there are staff who are committed to providing the best possible care despite appalling shortages.

It is obvious that people with advanced HIV disease do need medical and nursing care and are highly dependent on others. Clearly, if there is no new money provided to care for the increasing numbers and to train carers and health care workers, many will die in pain, isolation and distress, with carers feeling unsupported and desperate.

Attitudes and possibilities

For a person with AIDS the feeling of rejection by society is a devastating experience. Rejection is not always the result of judgement and censure on moral grounds, or because of a misguided fear of contracting the disease. Often it occurs because family members, friends and neighbours do not know how to cope with a young person who is dying. They feel awkward and embarrassed and at a loss for words, and therefore withdraw from the person who most needs their love and friendship.

(Williams, 1991)

Most patients, their families and friends need to be able to talk to someone about how they are feeling. They need information about what to expect and guidance on how they can help themselves and others. People trained in counselling have much to offer these families, as do religious leaders and pastoral care workers.

It is important for people with AIDS and their families to maintain or be given a sense of hope. If they feel accepted and have hope they will have a greater ability to cope with problems as they arise, and to live positively.

As has been said before, there is never 'nothing that can be done', and health carers can do much to assist in the maintenance of hope:

- care for the patients in an atmosphere of love and acceptance
- offer counselling
- help the patients to make the most of each day as it comes
- encourage the patient and family to have events to look forward to, e.g. visitors, small celebrations, outings
- set short-term achievable goals
- work with the patient to make the best out of difficult situations
- give information and advice to individuals relating to behaviour and infection risks
- encourage the patient to live as normal a life as possible

- encourage patients to look after themselves by eating nutritious food (when possible), taking plenty of rest and looking after their personal hygiene
- maintain a hopeful attitude as a carer.

Working with colleagues in Africa, we saw firsthand the difference the attitude of the health care professional can make to people with AIDS. Doctors in some hospitals, feeling helpless in the face of having to give a diagnosis of AIDS and with little treatment to offer, may choose to opt out; or if they do, pass on their own sense of hopelessness and may not see the patients at all. This only reinforces the patients' sense of helplessness. The result of this attitude, and of its opposite was evident when visiting outpatient clinics during which in excess of 180 patients might be seen in an afternoon. One doctor who was clearly depressed and feeling hopeless himself passed on this hopelessness to the patients he saw. He had good reason to feel helpless and hopeless, as he had very little medication to offer and most patients just received a handful of rice and some vitamins. However, at another clinic a doctor in just the same situation spent a couple of minutes encouraging the patients to get on with their lives despite a diagnosis of HIV. 'This news does not mean that your life is at an end; you have a lot of living left to do and I'm going to help you get on with it.' No more medication to offer, but those few words were better than a dose of medicine – the patient's look of hopelessness and fear went, to be replaced by a sense of hope and trust.

Counselling

Different models or understanding of the practice of counselling exist, and are much influenced by culture and society. In some countries it is very directive and involves the counsellor in identifying and, where possible, finding the solution to the problem. Where this expectation exists patients seek, and are often given advice by the expert; they do not expect to find their own solutions. A non-directive approach as practised in the West may not be what the patient is seeking, and may therefore be unacceptable. However, when a person has worked out his own solutions, with help by the counsellor to look at the available options, he is more likely to 'own' the decision and stick to it. For many, just being listened to and taken seriously will give them a sense of continuing worth and an ability to continue in spite of the problems.

Education and support for families

One of the greatest resources in developing countries is the extended family and efforts should be made to invest in these families.

A key to unlocking the problems where limited resources exist is education. Education should include health care professionals in both hospitals and community, teachers, religious and community leaders who can in turn cascade the information down to community health workers and volunteers, who can teach families about:

- AIDS – transmission, prevention and progression of HIV infection to symptomatic HIV and AIDS
- attitudes and behaviour
- how to care for someone with AIDS
- how to give emotional and spiritual support
- safe waste-disposal.

Where patients and their families are listened to, valued, supported, trained and assisted with activities of daily living as required, the quality of care can be greatly improved, even when other resources are in short supply.

Drama, role play and song are often the most effective tools of communication, and have already been extensively used in health education programmes throughout the world. Radio and television, too, should be exploited for their potential in reaching large audiences to increase knowledge and to change attitudes, not only in matters of prevention but also of care for ill people.

Community-based care programmes

In a regional workshop on community-based care in HIV/AIDS arranged in 1991 in Entebbe, Uganda, Dr C. Cameron, WHO Health Economist, made the following comment: 'While examination of financing issues can be a demanding task, there are already some encouraging indications concerning community-based care'.

Home-based care involves a great deal more than drug delivery and counselling, although these would usually be components of such a programme. It is clear that much of the care for people with HIV or AIDS will inevitably have to be based at home as hospitals are unable to cope with present workloads. Already a number of very impressive home based programmes have been developed and are well established, for example the integrated programme of care and prevention developed by the Salvation Army Hospital, Chikankata, Zambia, and the HIV clinic and Homecare programme set up by Nsambya Hospital, Kampala, in Uganda. These were initiated by, and are maintained from a hospital base.

The self-help organisation TASO started by Noerine Kaleeba in Uganda in 1987 is an example of what can be done when affected and infected people identify their own needs and start to deal with them together. TASO expanded rapidly and now has services which include counselling, medical and social support, with the head office in Kampala and six other centres along the trans-African highway in Uganda. It is supported by Action Aid.

TASO also runs a day centre where people with AIDS may meet, share a meal and other activities. A large number of orphans or children whose parents have AIDS are supported through primary school. Initially the home care provided simply counselling and social support, but now it also includes visits from medical personnel, and families are taught simple skills to care for the sick person.

TASO has also developed a community programme in response to requests from communities who wanted training, information and home care. The communities identify their own needs and priorities, and TASO provides supportive education and training.

The above examples, and that of UWESO (Uganda Women's Efforts to Save Orphans), provide excellent models from which to learn about effective approaches to care in the community for people with AIDS and their families and carers. UWESO, through its many local branch committees, encourages income-generating projects to support widows and orphans.

Below are some options which have been shown to be effective to a greater or lesser degree and which may be considered as starting points. However, it may be remembered that initiatives which are entirely hospital-based or external to the communities, with periodic visits into hospital, are expensive and may tend to increase a sick person's sense of dependence and helplessness, however grateful he may be. On the other hand, when people or communities are encouraged to identify their own needs and to find their own solutions, with support and training as appropriate, they will retain or develop a sense of control and independence which is likely to be very much more productive.

AIDS deepens the poverty level of people with AIDS and their families, and therefore severely limits what the families or communities can provide at home. Income generating schemes, with appropriate training, will therefore often be an essential part of enabling and empowering people to remain independent with a sense of self-respect and dignity. Some options which do not necessarily require large resources, other than human commitment and effort and probably transport, could include the following:

- Discharge planning with families and follow-up of patients admitted to hospital in their own homes.
- Counselling and pastoral support provided through trained volunteers in clinics and health centres or other meeting places such as churches.

- Training of community based health workers to include support for people with AIDS and their families.
- Basic training for families in simple nursing skills or the administration of certain medications or therapies, such as oral rehydration.
- Training for community volunteers, religious leaders and pastoral carers to provide practical care, and emotional and spiritual support.
- Simple symptom control training for nurses and doctors visiting patients at home.
- Day centres in villages or town set up in community centres or churches with good access to provide a meeting place for social and therapeutic support for people with AIDS and their carers.
- Visiting home care teams of trained nurses, doctors, social workers or counsellors as appropriate, to support and train more local community based carers.
- Income generation schemes with training and support for small business ventures through, for example, a 'rolling loans' arrangement with a local bank.

Links should be developed with community services and groups, both governmental and voluntary, to build upon or integrate with existing networks of care or communication. In particular, where community based programmes exist, for example for tuberculosis or leprosy prevention and care, these may provide excellent entry points into communities.

Church or other religious groups, with their existing networks and support structures, or traditional societies should also provide effective means of communication and social and/or spiritual care.

Safe waste-disposal

This may be a problem in parts of the world where almost everything that is discarded from hospitals and clinics is dumped in an open accessible site. It is then recycled by scavengers who make a living by selling disposable needles and syringes. These should be made safe by being flushed through, then discarded into a container (eg. glass bottle) with 1:10 bleach solution (or other effective disinfectant). The container with its contents may be buried, or incinerated if possible. Blood-stained cloths, if not being washed (in water above 60°C) and re-used, should be incinerated if possible. In the home, boiling such cloths will ensure disinfection. If they are being discarded, burning them would be the safest method of disposal.

Table 15. A basic home care kit

If available	Gloves, plasters, soap, sheets, rubber sheet, plastic aprons
For pain and pyrexias	
Headaches, general aches and pains, fever	Aspirin Paracetamol Codeine phosphate
Joint and bone pains, inflammation and pressure sores	Brufen Indomethacin (phenylbutazone)
For diarrhoea	Codeine phosphate Loperamide Kaolin mixture ORS
For nausea and vomiting	Stemetil Cyclizine Metoclopramide
For skin problems	
Fungal infections	Canestan cream Gentian violet paint
Itching without infection	Eurax (Crotamiton cream) Hydrocortisone cream Betnovate cream
Bacterial infections	Antibiotic tablets
Scabies	Sulphur ointment (or sim.) Benzyl benzoate, lorexane, malathion
Herpes simplex and zoster	Acyclovir tabs. and cream (if available)
For infections	
Chest and urinary tract infections; skin infection abscesses; some diarrhoeas respond to Septrin or metronidazole	Septrin/Bactrim Tetracycline Erythromycin Penicillin V Metronidazole
Suspected meningitis (should be hospitalised)	Chloramphenicol
Malaria Eye infections	Chloroquine Tetracycline eye ointment

Table 15. Cont'd

Oral or vaginal candidiasis	Nystatin susp/tabs.
	Gentian violet paint
	Clotrimazole tabs
For anxiety and agitation	Diazepam
	Chlorpromazine
For allergies	Piriton
	Phenergan
Miscellaneous	Ferrous sulphate
	Multivitamins
	Ventolin
	Codeine cough linctus

Note: see also Chapter 6 for symptom control details

References

Living with AIDS in the Community. WHO (1992).

Merson, M.H. (1993). *The HIV/AIDS Pandemic – Global Spread and Global Response.* (1993) IXth International conference on AIDS, Berlin.

Report of the World Health Organisation/Commonwealth Secretariat Regional Workshop on HIV/AIDS Community-based Care and Control, Entebbe, Uganda, 1991.

Williams, G. (ed.) (1991) Strategies for Hope. Action Aid, London.
No.1. From Hope to fear: Aids Care and Prevention at Chikankata Hospital, Zambia (1990)
No.2. Living Positively with AIDS: TASO (1990)
No.3. AIDS Management: An Integrated Approach (1990)
No.5. AIDS Orphans: A Community Perspective from Tanzania (1991)
No.6. The Caring Community: Coping with AIDS in Uganda (1991)

Further reading

References cited in the text are given at the end of the particular chapter.

Clinical and nursing

AIDS

Adler, M.W. (Ed.) 1987). *ABC of AIDS*. British Medical Journal, London.
Farthing, C. (1986). *A Colour Atlas of AIDS*. Wolfe Publishing Ltd, London.
Farthing, C., Brown, S., Staughton, R. (1988). *A Colour Atlas of AIDS and HIV Disease*, second edition. Wolfe Publishing Ltd, London.
Friedman-Kein, A.E. (1988). *Colour Atlas of AIDS*. W.B. Saunders, London.
Miller, D., Webber, J., Cress, J. (1986). *The Management of AIDS patients*. Macmillan, Basingstoke.
Pratt, R. (1991). *AIDS: A Strategy for Nursing Care*, third edition. Edward Arnold, London.
Rosenblum, M.L., Levy, R.M., Bredesen, D.W. (1988), *AIDS and the Nervous System*. Raven Press, New York.
Royal College of Nursing (1986). *Nursing Guidelines on the Management of Patients in Hospital and the Community suffering from AIDS*. Scutari Press, London.
Youle, M., Farthing, C., Clarbour, J., Wade, P. (1988), *AIDS: Therapeutics in HIV Disease*. Churchill Livingstone, Edinburgh.

General

Bates, T.D., Duncan, W., Ellis, H., Sikora, K. *et al.* (Eds). *Clinical Oncology. Contemporary Palliation of Difficult Symptoms*, Balliere, London.
Manning, M. (1984). *The Hospice Alternative. Living with Dying*. Souvenir Press, London.
Munley, A. (1983). *The Hospice Alternative. A new context for death and dying*. Basic Books, London.

156   **Further reading**

Swerdlow, M. and Ventafridda, V. (Eds). (1987). *Cancer Pain*. MTP Press Ltd, Lancaster, UK.
Twycross, R. and Lack, S. (1990). *Therapeutics in Terminal Cancer*, second edition. Churchill Livingstone, Edinburgh.

Social, counselling and pastoral issues

AIDS

Green, J. (1989). *Counselling in HIV infection and AIDS*. Blackwell Scientific Publications, Oxford,
Kirkpatrick, B. (1988). *AIDS: Sharing the Pain*, Darton, Longman and Todd, London.
Kubler-Ross, E. (1987). *AIDS: The Ultimate Challenge*. Macmillan, Basingstoke.
Marcetti, A. and Lunn, S. (1993) *A Place of Growth*. Darton, Longman and Todd Ltd. London.
Miller, D. (1987). *Living with AIDS and HIV*. Macmillan, Basingstoke.
Miller, R. and Bor, R. (1988) *AIDS: A Guide to Clinical Counselling*. Science Press, London.
Oyler, C. and Oyler, J. (1988). *Go Toward the light*. Harper and Rowe, London.
Shilts, R. (1988). *And the Band Played On*. Penguin Books, Harmondsworth, Middlesex.

General

Ainsworth-Smith, I. and Speck, P. (1982). *Letting Go*. Society for the Promotion of Christian Knowledge, London.
Cassidy, S. (1988). *Sharing the Darkness*. Darton, Longman and Todd, London.
Foskett, J. and Lyall, D. (1988). *Helping the Helpers – Supervision and Pastoral Care*. Society for the Promotion of Christian Knowledge, London.
Government White Paper, (1989). *Caring for People – Community Care in the Next Decade and Beyond*. CM849. HMSO, London.
Kubler-Ross, E. (1982). *Living with Death and Dying*. Souvenir Press, London.
McGilloway, O. and Myco, F. (1985). *Nursing and Spiritual Care*. Harper and Row, London.
Neuberger, J. (1987). *Caring for Dying People of Different Faiths*. Austen Cornish, London.
Saunders, C. Hospice and Palliative Care (1990) Edward Arnold, London.
Saunders, C. *Beyond the Horizon* (1990) Darton, Longman and Todd, London.
Speck, R. (1988). *Being There – Pastoral Care in Time of Illness*. Society for the Promotion of Christian Knowledge, London.

Women and children's issues

Claxton, R. and Harrison, A. (1990). *Caring for Children with HIV and AIDS*. Edward Arnold, London.

Richardson, D. (1989). *Women and the AIDS Crisis*, second edition. Pandora Press, London.

Women with HIV and AIDS (1993). (Ed.) Johnson M. and Johnstone F. Churchill Livingstone, Edinburgh.

Drug misuse/abuse and AIDS

Advisory Council on the Misuse of Drugs (1984). *Report*. HMSO, London.

Advisory Council on the Misuse of Drugs (1988). *AIDS and Drug Misuse*, HMSO, London.

Banks, A. and Waller, T.A.M. (1988). *Drug Misuse – A Practical Handbook for General Practitioners*. Blackwell Scientific Publications, Oxford.

Brettle, R.P. (1987). *Evidence to the Working Party on AIDS and Drug Misuse*. Advisory Council on Misuse of Drugs, HMSO, London.

Brettle, R.P., Bisset, K., Burns, S. *et al.* (1987). Human immunodeficiency virus and drug abuse: the Edinburgh experience. *British Medical Journal*, **294**, 421–4.

Bulkin, W., Brown, L., Fraioli, D. (1988). Hospice care for the intravenous drug user – AIDS patients in a skilled nurse facility. *Journal of Acquired Immuno-deficiency*, **1**, 375–80.

Croft-White, C., and Rayner, G. (1993). *Assessment and Care Management for Alcohol and Drug Misusers:* Advice to Local Authorities. SCODA and Alcohol Concern, London.

Robertson, J.R., Bucknill, A.B.V., Wellsby, P.D. *et al.* (1986). An epidemic of AIDS related virus (HTLV-III/LAV) injection amongst intravenous drug abusers in Scottish general practice. *British Medical Journal*, **292**, 527–30.

Robertson, A.R. (1987), *Heroin, AIDS and Society*, Hodder and Stoughton, Sevenoaks, Kent.

Siegel, L. (Ed.) (1988) *AIDS and Substance Abuse*, Haworth Press Inc., New York.

UK Health Department. *Guidance for Clinical Health Care Workers: Protection Against Infection with HIV and Hepatitis Viruses*. HMSO, London.

Appendix 1

Useful addresses in the UK (correct in August 1994)

Action Aid
Hamlyn House
Archway
London N19 5PG
Telephone (071) 281 4101
Fax (071) 272 0899

AIDS Care Education and Training (ACET)
PO Box 3693
London SW15 2BQ
Telephone (081) 780 0400 (General); (081) 780 0455 (Home Care only)
Fax (081) 780 0450

Body Positive
51B Philbeach Gardens
London SW5 9EB
Telephone (071) 835 1045
Fax (071) 373 5237

British Humanist Association
47 Theobald's Road
London WC1X 8SP
Telephone (071) 430 0908

The British Red Cross
Beautycare and Cosmetic Camouflage Department
National Headquarters
9 Grosvenor Crescent
London SW1X 7EJ
Telephone (071) 235 5454
(Beautycare organisers are available at local county branches.)

Cruse Bereavement Care
Cruse House
126 Sheen Road
Richmond
Surrey TW9 1UR
Telephone (081) 940 4818

The London Lighthouse
111–117 Lancaster Road
London W11 1QT
Telephone (071) 792 1200
Fax (071) 229 1258 (Main office)

Mainliners
PO Box 125
London SW9 8EF
Telephone (071) 737 3141

Mildmay Mission Hospital
Hackney Road
London E2 7NA
Telephone (071) 739 2331
Fax (071) 729 5361

Positive Partners/ Positively Children
The Annexe
Jan Rebane Centre
12–14 Thornston Street
London SW9 0BL
Telephone (071) 738 7333

Positively Women
5 Sebastian Street
London EC1V 0HE
Telephone (071) 490 5501 (Admin)
(071) 490 5515 (Clients)

Teaching Aids at Low Cost (TALC)
P.O. Box 49
St Albans
Herts. AL1 4AX
Telephone 0727 853869
Fax 0727 846852

The Terrence Higgins Trust (THT)
52–54 Grays Inn Road
London WC1X 8JU
Telephone (071) 831 0330
Helpline (071) 242 1010 (12 noon – 10pm daily)
Legal (071) 405 2381 (7–9pm Mon & Wed)
Fax (071) 242 0121

UK NGO AIDS Consortium for the Third World
Fenner Brockway House
37/39 Great Guildford Street
London SE1 OES, UK
Telephone (44 71) 401 8231
Fax (44 71) 401 2124

Appendix 2

Checklist of benefits available for people with AIDS/HIV in the UK (1994)

Employed or Self-employed *Fit for Work*	Family Credit Housing Benefit Social Fund – Crisis Loans Income Support Disabled Working Allowance Child Benefit One Parent Benefit
Employed or Self-employed *Unfit for Work*	Statutory Sick Pay (SSP) Sickness Benefits Invalidity Benefit (after 28 weeks) Income Support Housing Benefit Disabled Living Allowance Social Fund Payments
Not Employed (Have sufficient National Insurance Contributions) *Fit for Work*	Unemployment Benefit Income Support Housing Benefit Disabled Living Allowance Social Fund Payments
Not Employed (Have sufficient National Insurance Contributions) *Unfit for Work*	Sickness Benefit Invalidity Benefit (after 28 weeks) Income Support Housing Benefit Disabled Living Allowance Social Fund Payments

Not Employed (Insufficient contributions paid) e.g. people who have not worked for some time	Income Support Housing Benefits Disabled Living Allowance Social Fund Payments
Not Employed (Insufficient Contributions paid) *Unfit for Work*	Income Support Severe Disablement Allowance (after 28 weeks) Housing Benefits Disabled Living Allowance Social Fund payments

Child Benefit for all
One Parent Benefit (if applicable)
Council Tax Benefit for all
(All dependent on whether they meet the criteria.)

Index